/ 95

HEALTHIER EATING

AND LIVING WITH CANCER

HEALTHIER EATING

AND LIVING WITH CANCER

KAREN JUNG

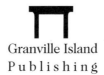

Granville Island
Publishing

LIBRARY AND ARCHIVES CANADA CATALOGUING IN PUBLICATION

Jung, Karen 1960–

Healthier eating and living with cancer / written by Karen Jung.
Includes index.

ISBN 978–1–894694–57–5

1. Cancer—Diet therapy—Recipes.
2. Cancer—Treatment—Complications—Diet therapy—Recipes.
     I. Title.
     II. Title: Healthier eating and living with cancer.

RC271.D52J85 2008   641.5'631   C2007–907475–8

Granville Island Publishing Ltd.
212–1656 Duranleau St., Granville Island
Vancouver BC · Canada · V6H 3S4
1–800–688–0320
info@granvilleislandpublishing.com
www.granvilleislandpublishing.com

First Published March 2008
Printed in Canada

08 09 10 ♦ 3 2 1

I dedicate this cookbook in memory of my beloved husband and best friend, Jeff.

The writing and publication of this book would not have been possible without his encouragement.

Acknowledgements

First of all, I want to especially thank my mother, Mei, and my brothers and sisters for all their wonderful support of Jeff and I over the years. I will always remember their words of encouragement and tremendous help in every possible way during Jeff's illness.

Next, I want to thank Dr. Brian Thiessen, Neuro Oncologist at the BC Cancer Agency in Vancouver, for reviewing my manuscript and offering me his invaluable advice and support.

Also, special thanks to my family and friends who tested my recipes endlessly over the years and offered their constructive feedback.

Last but not least, many thanks to Jo Blackmore, my publisher, for sharing her publishing and marketing expertise and guiding me through the entire book publishing process.

CONTENTS

Introduction

I was initially inspired to write this book with the encouragement of my husband, Jeff. I also wanted to help other people living with cancer or life-threatening illnesses to prepare healthier meals. A proper diet is crucial for everyone, but especially for people undergoing cancer treatments.

Jeff's and my lives changed suddenly when he was diagnosed with cancer. We made some serious lifestyle changes, including our eating habits, for the long journey ahead together. Jeff had to be more dependent on me for his daily needs. I wanted to help him as much as possible with his recovery from ongoing cancer treatments. It was a difficult time but I will always remember how his illness reinforced our deep love for each other. We became much closer as husband and wife. Jeff and I always enjoyed cooking and eating together. We often surprised each other with new creations and recipes. He was very adept at making meals from whatever was in the refrigerator. I found the process of developing new recipes fun and exciting, so our combined talents served us well.

It is not uncommon that during chemotherapy treatment a person's appetite and taste for certain foods changes. The challenge is to prepare meals that remain palatable with changes in health conditions and to find a variety of foods that help maintain or increase weight.

I researched cancer-fighting and antioxidant-abundant foods before developing a more structured diet to fit with my husband's cancer treatments. He took a strong interest in the planning of his daily meals especially as his health condition changed. He was the ultimate tester for the recipes for my cookbook. All recipes have been tested repeatedly on others too, to seek additional feedback.

During cancer treatments and post-treatment recovery, especially on days when eating was most challenging, we included high-energy and high-protein foods. High-fibre and potassium-rich foods were used on days of reduced physical activity and to counteract the side effects of prescribed chemotherapy and anti-nausea medications. Including lower-fat foods and monitoring bad fat intake — especially foods with trans fats and some saturated fats — was paramount. Foods abundant in antioxidants for cell repair, possible cancer prevention and premature aging were encouraged. Calcium-enriched foods to offset the reduced bone density associated with prescribed steroid medications were also used. Meals in this cookbook were designed with an emphasis on all of these factors.

It is very important to enjoy a variety of foods daily from the four food groups in *Eating Well with Canada's Food Guide*. The four food groups are vegetables and fruit, grain products, milk and alternatives, and meat and alternatives. Recommended daily servings are based on age and gender.

Eating properly, eating regularly and eating on time are crucial during cancer treatments. A combination of smaller meals, larger meals and/or frequent snacks every day is essential. Offer back-up food choices and selections as food tastes will change from time to time. The recipes in this book helped to prevent weight loss and nausea during Jeff's cancer treatments.

Cooking meals at home, including baking from scratch, is ideal. This allows you to have control over the quality of ingredients, amount and type of fats, sodium level and calorie intake. It is smart to take control of your food intake, which in turn impacts cholesterol levels.

This collection of over 160 easy-to-make recipes, with step-by-step instructions, is user-friendly even for newer cooks and the recipes are practical for any busy household. There are recipes in this book that will appeal to even more selective eaters. Some of the recipes are culturally diverse and suitable for both Western and Eastern tastes. All ingredients are available in supermarkets or in Asian and ethnic sections of stores. Most ingredients are affordable even for those with large families and a fixed budget. I encourage you to use all-natural dried fruits and unsalted nuts and fresh herbs and spices as much as possible. From our personal experience, higher quality baking and cooking ingredients make all the difference in your outcome.

Please note that this cookbook is not intended to replace any medical or nutritional advice. It reflects our experience only. Moreover, please consult with your treating physician, oncologist and/or nutritionist regarding your own individual situation as each person's health and side effects during cancer treatments is different.

Antioxidants and Cancer Prevention

Antioxidants are substances that protect cells from damage caused by unstable molecules known as free radicals. Free radicals are molecules with missing electrons. They steal electrons from other complete molecules by invading the healthy tissues of the body and killing the formerly healthy cells in the process. Free radicals may cause cancer. Antioxidants keep cells healthy, stabilize free radicals and reduce the risk of cancer.

Foods that are abundant in antioxidants include various fruits and vegetables, as well as nuts, grains, some lean meats, poultry and fish.

Beta-carotene, lutein, lycopene, selenium and vitamins A, C and E are common antioxidant nutrients. Beta-carotene is found in many orange-coloured fruits and vegetables such as apricots, cantaloupe, mangoes, carrots, squash and sweet potatoes. Lutein is abundant in green, leafy vegetables such as kale and spinach. Lycopene-rich fruits include apricots, blood oranges, watermelon, tomatoes and tomato products. Rice, wheat and Brazil nuts are high in selenium. Vitamin A is found in foods such as carrots, sweet potatoes, milk, egg yolks and mozzarella cheese. Vitamin C is found in citrus fruits, vegetables, cereals, beef, poultry and fish. Vitamin E is found in foods such as almonds, wheat germ, mangoes and broccoli.

Foods & Spices Abundant in Antioxidants (Cancer-Fighting Compounds) in this Book

Fruits	Vegetables	Other	Spices
Apples (with skin)	Asparagus	Almonds	Curries
Apricots	Black Beans	Eggs (yolks)	Garlic
Avocados	Broccoli	Extra Virgin Olive Oil	Ginger
Blackberries	Cabbage	Flax Seeds	
Blueberries	Carrots (with skin)	Milk	
Cantaloupe	Cauliflower	Mozzarella Cheese	
Cranberries	Celery	Oats	
Grapes (purple & red)	Onions	Rice (brown)	
Lemons	Peppers	Salmon	
Mangoes	Potatoes	Tofu	
Oranges	Red Kidney Beans	Tomato Sauce	
Pineapple	Shiitake Mushrooms	Wheat Germ	
Plums (purple)	Spinach	Yogurt	
Raspberries	Split Peas		
Strawberries	Squash		
Tomatoes	Sweet Potatoes		
Watermelon	Swiss Chard/ Bok Choy		
	Yams		

Foods High in Fibre

Fruits	Vegetables	Other
Apples (with skin)	Asparagus	Almonds
Apricots	Bean Sprouts	Applesauce
Avocados	Beans	Beef
Bananas	Broccoli	Bran Cereal & Raisins
Blueberries	Cabbage	Bran Muffin
Cantaloupe	Carrots	Cheese
Cherries	Cauliflower	Chicken
Figs	Celery	Coconut
Fruit Juices (apple, grape & orange)	Corn	Eggs
Grapes (black & red)	Cucumber	English Muffin
Honeydew	Green Peas	Fish
Oranges	Kidney Beans	Flax Seeds
Pears	Lettuce	Hot Dog Bun
Pineapple	Mushrooms	Macaroni
Plums	Onions	Milk
Raisins	Peppers	Peanut Butter
Raspberries	Potatoes (with skin)	Peanuts
Strawberries	Snow Peas	Pork
Tomatoes	Spinach	Rice
Watermelon	Split Peas	Rye Bread
	Squash	Spaghetti
	Sweet Potatoes (with skin)	Strawberry Yogurt
	Swiss Chard/Bok Choy	Tofu
	Zucchini	Tortilla (flour)
		Turkey
		Walnuts

Foods Rich in Potassium

Fruits	Vegetables	Other
Apricots	Broccoli	Almonds
Avocados	Cabbage	Bran Cereals
Bananas	Carrots	Cashews
Cantaloupe	Kidney Beans	Chocolate (dark)
Dried Fruits (apricots, figs & raisins)	Mushrooms	Milk
Fruit Juice (orange)	Potatoes	Molasses
Honeydew	Spinach	Peanuts
Oranges	Split Peas	Strawberry Yogurt
Tomatoes	Squash (orange flesh)	
	Sweet Potatoes	
	Swiss Chard/Bok Choy	

Popular Breakfast Menus

1. Apple juice, Homemade Belgian Waffles with maple syrup, pork sausages (skin removed)/ Scrambled Eggs with ketchup, clementines

2. Cranberry juice/grape juice, Spinach and Cheese Pancake, 1% salt bacon slices, watermelon chunks/cherry tomatoes

3. Orange juice with calcium, strawberry yogurt, skim milk, whole wheat toast with peanut butter

4. Orange juice with calcium, strawberry yogurt, Texas-Size Banana Blueberry Muffin/Giant Blueberry Muffin/Large Blueberry Bran Muffin

5. Orange juice with calcium, strawberry yogurt, Large Blueberry Bran Muffin, banana

6. Orange juice with calcium, strawberry yogurt, bran cereal with raisins & skim milk/rye toast with peanut butter, watermelon chunks/honeydew chunks

7. Orange juice with calcium, strawberry yogurt, soft-boiled eggs, Homemade Belgian Waffles with maple syrup

8. Orange juice with calcium, strawberry yogurt, Spinach and Cheese Pancake, tater gems

9. Orange juice with calcium, Scrambled Eggs, tater gems with ketchup

10. Wild blueberry cocktail, Spinach and Cheese Pancake, deli turkey breast slices

11. Banana Blueberry Smoothies, rye toast with peanut butter/Large Blueberry Bran Muffin

12. Skim milk, Scrambled Eggs, 1% salt bacon slices, herbed potatoes with ketchup/toasted English muffin with peanut butter

13. Bran with raisins cereal bar, banana

14. English muffin with marmalade, Scrambled Eggs with ketchup, pork sausages (skin removed), garden tomato slices

15. English muffin with peanut butter, 1% salt bacon slices

16. Homemade Belgian Waffles with maple syrup/1% salt bacon slices, soft-boiled eggs

17. Rye toast with peanut butter, fried eggs with extra virgin olive oil, pork sausages (skin removed)

18. Rye toast with peanut butter, Scrambled Eggs, deli turkey breast slices

Breakfast Menu Suggestions

Juices/ Smoothies	Milk/ Yogurt	Breads/ Cereals	Eggs	Meats	Vegetables	Fruits
Apple juice	Skim milk	Homemade Belgian Waffles with maple syrup	Fried eggs with extra virgin olive oil	1% salt bacon slices	Herbed potatoes	Banana
Cranberry juice	Strawberry yogurt	Spinach and Cheese Pancake	Scrambled Eggs with ketchup	Italian sausage	Tater gems with ketchup	Clementines
Grape juice		Texas-Size Banana Blueberry Muffin	Soft-boiled eggs	Pork sausages (skin removed)		Honeydew chunks
Orange juice with calcium		Giant Blueberry Muffin		Turkey breast slices (deli)		Watermelon chunks
Wild blueberry cocktail		Large Blueberry Bran Muffin				Cherry tomatoes
Banana Blueberry Smoothies		Bran cereal with raisins & skim milk				Garden tomato slices
		Bran with raisins cereal bar				
		Rye toast with peanut butter				
		English muffin with peanut butter				
		Whole wheat toast with peanut butter				

Lunch Menu Suggestions

Juices	Yogurt	Breads	Eggs	Meats	Rice/Salads/Vegetables	Fruits
Apple juice		Karen's 15-Inch Deluxe Pizza slices				Banana
Apple juice		Spinach & cheese pizza			Greek salad	Watermelon chunks
Apple juice		Chicken Salad on Toasted Rye			Greek salad/ green salad with avocado chunks	Honeydew chunks
Apple juice				Grilled sirloin steak with garlic & black pepper	Potato & cheese perogies, green salad with avocado chunks	
Apple juice		Grilled Turkey and Swiss Sandwiches			Sliced dill pickles	Mandarin oranges
Apple juice				Bavarian smokies	Cheddar broccoli pasta shells	Honeydew chunks
Cranberry juice		Karen's 15-Inch Deluxe Pizza slices				Fresh blueberries
Grape juice		Deli chicken breast slices on Kaiser buns				Roma tomato halves
Orange juice with calcium	Strawberry yogurt	Rye toast with peanut butter				Honeydew chunks & prunes
Wild blueberry cocktail		Grilled Fajita chicken breast & Swiss cheese on rye			Sliced dill pickles & pickled asparagus spears	
		Chicken Salad on Toasted Rye			Garden green beans/potato salad	

Lunch Menu Suggestions (cont.)

Juices	Yogurt	Breads	Eggs	Meats	Rice/Salads/Vegetables	Fruits
Wild blueberry cocktail		All-beef hot dogs on hoagie buns				Watermelon chunks
			Poached Eggs on English Muffins			Garden tomato slices
		English muffin with marmalade jam	Scrambled Eggs		Herbed potatoes/tater gems	Clementines
			Scrambled eggs with diced chicken breast	Boiled pork sausages (skin removed)	Herbed potatoes/tater gems	Watermelon chunks
			Chicken breast & Swiss cheese omelette			
		Toasted English muffin with peanut butter	Sun-dried tomato Turkey and Swiss Omelette		Baby carrots	
		Grilled cheese, tomato & bacon on rye			Sliced dill pickles & pickled asparagus spears	
		Salmon Salad on Toasted Rye/English muffins			Potato salad	Honeydew chunks/ black plum
		Grilled turkey breast & Swiss cheese on rye			Sliced dill pickles & potato salad/ Greek salad	Cantaloupe slices
		Turkey breast & tomato on whole wheat sub			Celery sticks	Raspberries

Lunch Menu Suggestions (cont.)

Juices	Yogurt	Breads	Eggs	Meats	Rice/Salads/Vegetables	Fruits
				Deli chicken breast slices	Garden green beans, microwave squash/ sweet potato, microwave potato half	Garden tomato slices
				Dark and Delicious Homemade Chili	Tossed Green Salad with Flax Seed Oil	
				Honey and Garlic Pork Spareribs	Rice, snap peas & green salad/broccoli	
				Teriyaki Pork Loin Chop	Sweet potato, baby potatoes, peas/broccoli & butternut squash/ Cheddar broccoli pasta salad	
				Karen's Hearty Shepherd's Pie	Quick Caesar Salad/Greek salad	
				Roast Honey and Spice Turkey drumstick	Microwave yam & potato half	

Dinner Menu Suggestions

Juices/Milk	Breads	Salads	Meats/ Pastas	Rice/Tofu	Vegetables	Fruits
			Karen's 15-Inch Deluxe Pizza slices		Green beans, snap peas	
		Quick Caesar Salad	Spinach Lasagne			
			Rotini pasta twists/ spaghetti/ penne with tomato & meat sauce		Steamed broccoli	
		Green salad	Beef tortellini with tomato & meat sauce		Garden green beans	
Cranberry juice			Chicken tortellini with tomato & meat sauce		Snow peas/ yam & steamed broccoli	
		Green salad/ Quick Caesar Salad	Seafood Fettuccine Alfredo		Steamed asparagus spears	Garden cherry tomatoes
	Whole wheat bun		Easy Beef Stew			Avocado half
			Karen's Cabbage Rolls		Steamed broccoli	
Skim milk		Green salad with avocado chunks/Greek salad	Karen's Hearty Shepherd's Pie			Sliced Bosch pear (peeled & cored)
Apple juice/ Skim milk		Green salad with avocado chunks & teaspoon of flax seed oil/ vinaigrette coleslaw & potato salad/ Greek salad	Microwave chicken breast with garlic, salt & black pepper		Microwave potato half, snow peas/ green beans/ sultan squash, steamed broccoli & sweet potato/ Shanghai bok choy	Sliced garden tomato/Roma tomatoes/ honeydew chunks
		Green salad	Spicy Almond Chicken		Microwave potato & yam	Sliced garden tomato

Dinner Menu Suggestions (cont.)

Juices/Milk	Breads	Salads	Meats/Pastas	Rice/Tofu	Vegetables	Fruits
Apple juice		Greek salad/ green salad with teaspoon of flax seed oil	Oven-baked breaded chicken breast/legs		Sui choy (Napa cabbage)/ microwave yam half & sweet potato	Avocado half
			Honey Garlic Chicken, cheese & potato perogies		Snap peas	
		Quick Caesar Salad	Steamed chicken breast		Cheesy scalloped potatoes, East Meets West Vegetarian Casserole	Grape tomatoes
Apple juice		Green salad	Oven-baked Canadian Northern whitefish		Cheesy scalloped potatoes, snap peas/yam, microwave potato half & steamed broccoli/ cauliflower & sweet potato	Sliced D'Anjou pear (peeled & cored)
		Green salad	Braised mackerel steak with black bean garlic sauce	Braised tofu cubes in black bean sauce	Green beans	
			Steamed snapper fillet with extra virgin olive oil, black pepper, sliced ginger & green onion, cheese & potato perogies		Snow peas/ cheesy scalloped potatoes & steamed broccoli/gai lan/bok choy/ Chinese Napa cabbage/ microwave potato, sultan squash, green beans, sweet potato/green peas	Garden cherry tomatoes

Dinner Menu Suggestions (cont.)

Juices/Milk	Breads	Salads	Meats/ Pastas	Rice/Tofu	Vegetables	Fruits
Skim milk		Green salad with avocado chunks	Oven-baked pink salmon		Steamed broccoli, sweet potato half, baby potatoes/yam & microwave potato half	
		Green salad/ potato salad	Half tin of sockeye salmon, macaroni & cheese/ rigatoni with tomato & meat sauce		Green beans/ steamed broccoli/ sultan squash, baby potatoes & green peas	
Skim milk			Glazed Whole Boneless Ham slices, potato & cheese perogies		Sautéed shiitake mushrooms with oyster sauce, steamed broccoli/sui choy (Napa cabbage)	Sliced D'Anjou pear (peeled & cored)
			Roast pork tenderloin	Tofu with mixed vegetables & black bean garlic sauce	Microwave potato, sweet potato, green beans/bok choy (Swiss chard) & Yukon Gold potatoes	
Cranberry juice		Greek salad/ green salad with teaspoon of flax seed oil	Teriyaki Pork Loin Chop, potato & cheese perogies	Boiled rice, tofu with black bean sauce	Steamed broccoli/ squash/ microwave potato half & sweet potato/ pickled asparagus spears	Sliced tomato
Apple juice		Greek salad, green salad	Grilled lamb chop with mint sauce, macaroni & cheese		Steamed broccoli/ microwave potato half & sweet potato	Avocado half with teaspoon of lemon juice

Dinner Menu Suggestions (cont.)

Juices/Milk	Breads	Salads	Meats/Pastas	Rice/Tofu	Vegetables	Fruits
Apple juice/ Cranberry juice		Green salad/ Greek salad	Honey and Garlic Pork Spareribs		Sautéed bean sprouts/ microwave potato half, squash, steamed cauliflower/ broccoli, sweet potato/ green beans	Sliced tomato/ D'Anjou pear (peeled & cored)
			Sweet and Sour Pork	Boiled rice	Gai lan/ steamed broccoli/ cauliflower/ green beans/ snap peas	
		Green salad, potato salad/ Greek salad	Grilled pork chop		Steamed broccoli/ green beans/ butternut squash	Sliced yellow tomatoes
Apple juice		Quick Caesar Salad/potato salad/green salad	Grilled sirloin steak with black pepper, macaroni & cheese		Steamed broccoli, microwave potato & yam/ sweet potato & green peas	
		Greek salad/ potato salad	Grilled T-bone steak		Squash, steamed broccoli/green beans	Garden cherry tomatoes
	Whole wheat bread		Roast beef with mushroom gravy		Brussels sprouts, squash, microwave potato half	
			Microwave turkey drumstick with garlic, salt, black pepper & oregano	Fried rice	Microwave potato/sweet potato/yam/ squash, snap peas/green beans	
	Easy Cheese Bread		Easy-To-Make Turkey Casserole		Snap peas	

Snack Ideas

Juices/ Smoothies	Milk	Dips	Cheeses/ Crackers	Muffins	Cookies/ Brownies	Cakes/ Pies	Fruits/ Nuts
Aloe vera juice	Skim milk	Black Bean dip with corn tortilla chips	Easy Cheese Bread (toasted)	Banana Coconut Muffin	The Very Best Chunky Peanut Butter Cookie	The Very Best Blueberry Crumb Cake square	Apple (Granny Smith)
100% pure apple juice		Chunky salsa with organic corn tortilla chips/corn chips with flax seeds	Unsalted crackers	Banana Cranberry Muffin	Giant Double Chocolate Walnut Cookie	Apple pie slice	Apricots
½ cup apple juice + 1 tsp flax seed oil + ¼ cup water			50% less salt whole wheat crackers with Swiss Emmenthal cheese	Monster-Size Banana Raisin Bran Muffin	Oatmeal Cranberry Cookie	10-Inch Homemade Blueberry Pie slice	Banana
Cranberry juice			Melba sesame rounds with low-fat cream cheese and smoked salmon/ pickled herring fillets	Triple Berry Bran Muffin	Lower-Fat Oatmeal Raisin Cookie		Blackberries
Grape juice			Low-salt pretzel sticks				Blueberries
Wild blueberry cocktail					Chocolate Walnut Brownie		Cherries
Banana Blueberry Smoothie							Clementines
Banana Raspberry Smoothie							Grapes (black & green)

Snack Ideas (cont.)

Juices/ Smoothies	Milk	Dips	Cheeses/ Crackers	Muffins	Cookies/ Brownies	Cakes/ Pies	Fruits/ Nuts
Blueberry Smoothie							Honeydew chunks
Citrus Blueberry Smoothie							Mandarin orange
Strawberry Smoothie							Mango wedges
							Nectarine
							Orange
							Peach
							Pear (Bosch & D'Anjou)
							Pineapple wedges
							Plum (black)
							Prune Plums
							Raspberries
							Strawberries
							Watermelon chunks
							Dried Fruits (blueberries, cranberries, figs, mangoes, raisins)
							Fruit flavoured jelly powder
							Whole almonds

Recommended Recipes
During and After Cancer Treatments

	Breakfast	Lunch	Snack	Dinner	During Treatment	After Treatment
Smoothies						
Banana Blueberry Smoothies	●		●			●
Banana Raspberry Smoothies	●				●	●
Banana Strawberry Smoothies			●			●
Citrus Blueberry Smoothies			●			●
Strawberry Smoothies			●			●
Appetizers						
Beef and Black Bean Tortilla Chip Dip		●	●			●
Chicken Quesadillas		●		●		●
Guacamole			●			●
Hummus Dip			●			●
Karen's Crab-Stuffed Mushroom Caps			●			●
Karen's Nacho Chips		●	●			●
Tzatziki (Yogurt-Cucumber Dip)			●		●	●
Vegetarian Quesadillas		●	●	●	●	●
Cookies						
Chocolate Chunk Cookies			●		●	●
Date Spice Cookies			●		●	●

	Breakfast	Lunch	Snack	Dinner	During Treatment	After Treatment
Cookies (cont.)						
Giant Chocolate Chip Cookies			●		●	●
Giant Chocolate Chip Walnut Cookies			●		●	●
Giant Coconut Raisin Cranberry Oatmeal Cookies			●		●	●
Giant Double Chocolate Walnut Cookies			●		●	●
Giant Oatmeal Blueberry Cranberry Cookies			●		●	●
Giant Oatmeal Chocolate Chip Raisin Cookies			●		●	●
Giant Oatmeal Chocolate Cookies			●		●	●
Giant Oatmeal Cranberry Raisin Cookies			●		●	●
Hearty Oatmeal Spice Cookies			●		●	●
Jumbo Cranberry White Chocolate Oatmeal Cookies			●		●	●
Lower-Fat Cranberry Chocolate Oatmeal Cookies			●		●	●
Lower-Fat Oatmeal Raisin Cookies			●		●	●
Lower-Fat Triple Fruit Oatmeal Cookies			●		●	●
Monster-Size Chocolate Chip Raisin Walnut Cookies			●		●	●
The Very Best Chunky Peanut Butter Cookies			●		●	●
The Very Best Peanut Butter Chocolate Chunk Cookies			●		●	●
Muffins						
Banana Coconut Muffins			●		●	●
Banana Cranberry Muffins			●		●	●
Big Coconut Raisin Muffins			●		●	●
Carrot Raisin Walnut Muffins	●		●		●	●
Chocolate Chip Walnut Surprise Muffins			●		●	●

	Breakfast	Lunch	Snack	Dinner	During Treatment	After Treatment
Muffins (cont.)						
Cranberry Apple Walnut Spice Muffins			●		●	●
Crunchy Peanut Butter Surprise Muffins			●		●	●
Extra-Large Triple Berry Muffins			●		●	●
Giant Blueberry Muffins			●		●	●
Large Blueberry Bran Muffins	●		●		●	●
Mixed Berry Healthy Muffins	●		●		●	●
Monster-Size Banana Raisin Bran Muffins	●		●		●	●
Super Double Chocolate Walnut Muffins			●		●	●
Texas-Size Banana Blueberry Muffins			●		●	●
Texas-Size Banana Mixed Berry Muffins			●		●	●
Brownies						
Chocolate Walnut Brownies			●			●
Dark and Rich Brownies			●			●
Cakes						
Easy-To-Make Chocolate Cake			●			●
The Very Best Blueberry Crumb Cake			●		●	●
The Very Best Dark Chocolate Cake			●			●
Pies						
9-Inch Apple Pie			●		●	●
10-Inch Apple Pie			●		●	●
10-Inch Homemade Blackberry-Blueberry Pie			●		●	●
10-Inch Homemade Blueberry Pie			●		●	●

	Breakfast	Lunch	Snack	Dinner	During Treatment	After Treatment
Fruit Desserts						
Apple Crisp			●		●	●
Fresh Fruit Salad	●	●	●	●	●	●
Fruity Dessert			●		●	●
Mixed Fruit Dessert			●		●	●
Poached Allspice Pears			●			●
Eggs						
Boiled Eggs	●				●	●
Pickled Eggs			●			●
Poached Eggs on English Muffins	●				●	●
Scrambled Eggs	●				●	●
Turkey and Swiss Omelette	●	●			●	●
Pancakes & Waffles						
Blueberry Cornmeal Pancakes	●				●	●
Homemade Belgian Waffles	●				●	●
Spinach and Cheese Pancakes	●	●				●
Soups						
Chicken and Corn Soup				●		●
Crab Soup				●		●
Karen's Hot and Sour Soup				●		●
Split Pea Soup		●		●		●
Tomato Clam Chowder		●				●

	Breakfast	Lunch	Snack	Dinner	During Treatment	After Treatment

Stews

	Breakfast	Lunch	Snack	Dinner	During Treatment	After Treatment
Dark and Delicious Homemade Chili		●		●		●
Easy Beef Stew				●	●	●
Hungarian Goulash				●		●

Sandwiches

	Breakfast	Lunch	Snack	Dinner	During Treatment	After Treatment
Chicken Salad on Toasted Rye		●			●	●
Egg Salad Sandwiches		●			●	●
Grilled Cheese Sandwiches		●			●	●
Grilled Ham and Cheese Sandwiches		●			●	●
Grilled Turkey and Swiss Sandwiches		●			●	●
Hummus Alfalfa Pita Pockets		●				●
Salmon Salad on Toasted Rye		●			●	●
Shrimp and Avocado Croissants		●			●	●

Breads, Calzones & Pizzas

	Breakfast	Lunch	Snack	Dinner	During Treatment	After Treatment
Banana Bread			●		●	●
Easy Cheese Bread		●	●			●
Karen's 15-Inch Beef and Sausage Pizza		●				●
Karen's 15-Inch Deluxe Pizza		●				●
Karen's 15-Inch Ham and Pineapple Pizza		●				●
Karen's 15-Inch Ham and Shrimp Pizza		●				●
Karen's 15-Inch Turkey and Cheese Pizza		●				●
Pepperoni Calzones		●				●

	Breakfast	Lunch	Snack	Dinner	During Treatment	After Treatment
Salads						
Great Caesar Salad				●		●
Mexican Corn and Bean Salad				●		●
Potato and Egg Salad		●		●	●	●
Quick Caesar Salad				●		●
Quick Greek Salad		●		●		●
Spinach and Mandarin Salad				●	●	●
Super Spinach, Egg and Bacon Salad				●	●	●
Three Bean Salad				●		●
Tomato Salad				●		●
Tossed Green Salad		●		●	●	●
Tossed Green Salad with Flax Seed Oil		●		●	●	●
Tossed Salad with Citrus Dressing				●		●
Beef						
Curry and Black Bean Beef				●		●
Karen's Cabbage Rolls				●		●
Karen's Hearty Shepherd's Pie		●		●	●	●
Pork						
Glazed Whole Boneless Ham				●	●	●
Honey and Garlic Pork Spareribs				●		●
Karen's Curried Pork				●		●
Sweet and Sour Pork				●		●
Teriyaki Pork Loin Chops				●	●	●

	Breakfast	Lunch	Snack	Dinner	During Treatment	After Treatment

Chicken

	Breakfast	Lunch	Snack	Dinner	During Treatment	After Treatment
Asian Chicken and Egg over Rice		●			●	●
Asian Chicken Casserole				●		●
Asian Roast Chicken				●		●
Caribbean Jerk Chicken				●		●
Curried Tomato Chicken				●		●
Fried Chicken		●		●		●
Hawaiian Chicken				●		●
Honey Curry Chicken				●		●
Honey Garlic Chicken				●		●
Oven-Baked Spiced Chicken				●		●
Spanish Paella				●		●
Spicy Almond Chicken				●		●
Teriyaki Chicken Breast Fajitas		●		●	●	●

Turkey

	Breakfast	Lunch	Snack	Dinner	During Treatment	After Treatment
Easy-To-Make Turkey Casserole				●	●	●
Roast Honey and Spice Turkey				●		●
Spanish Turkey and Rice				●		●

Seafood

	Breakfast	Lunch	Snack	Dinner	During Treatment	After Treatment
Braised Shrimp with Vegetables				●	●	●
Prawns with Vegetables				●	●	●
Steamed Whole Tilapia Fish				●	●	●

	Breakfast	Lunch	Snack	Dinner	During Treatment	After Treatment
Tofu						
Asian Curried Tofu				●		●
Asian Spicy Tofu				●		●
Tofu with Crabmeat				●	●	●
Tofu with Mushrooms and Peas				●	●	●
Tofu with Oyster Sauce				●	●	●
Tofu with Pork				●		●
Tofu with Vegetables				●	●	●
Pasta						
Cheesy Rigatoni and Broccoli Casserole				●		●
Ham and Cheese Pasta Salad				●		●
Homemade Spaghetti Sauce				●		●
Macaroni and Cheese		●			●	●
Mixed Seafood Fettuccine				●		●
Pasta Meat Sauce				●		●
Seafood Fettuccine Alfredo				●		●
Seafood Lasagne				●		●
Spinach Lasagne				●	●	●
Vegetarian Pasta Salad				●		●

	Breakfast	Lunch	Snack	Dinner	During Treatment	After Treatment
Rice						
Chicken and Shrimp Fried Rice				●	●	●
Prawn, Crab and Avocado Sushi		●		●		●
Rice Casserole				●	●	●
Spanish Rice				●	●	●
Vegetables & Sauce						
Asparagus Spears with Flax Seed Oil				●		●
Curried Potatoes				●		●
Deep Fried Zucchini Sticks		●		●		●
East Meets West Vegetarian Casserole				●	●	●
Glazed Carrots				●	●	●
Lemon-Parsley Potatoes				●	●	●
Mashed Potatoes				●	●	●
Mashed Sweet Potato Bake				●	●	●
Mixed Vegetables with Cashew Nuts				●	●	●
Cheese Sauce				●		●

Jeff's Top 25 Favourites

1. Banana Blueberry Smoothies
2. Citrus Blueberry Smoothies
3. Strawberry Smoothies
4. Giant Double Chocolate Walnut Cookies
5. The Very Best Chunky Peanut Butter Cookies
6. Giant Oatmeal Cranberry Raisin Cookies
7. Texas-Size Banana Blueberry Muffins
8. Large Blueberry Bran Muffins
9. The Very Best Blueberry Crumb Cake
10. 10-Inch Homemade Blackberry-Blueberry Pie
11. Karen's 15-Inch Deluxe Pizza
12. Spinach and Cheese Pancakes
13. Homemade Belgian Waffles
14. Beef and Black Bean Tortilla Chip Dip
15. Karen's Crab-Stuffed Mushroom Caps
16. Salmon Salad on Toasted Rye
17. Great Caesar Salad
18. Tossed Green Salad with Flax Seed Oil
19. Super Spinach, Egg and Bacon Salad
20. Dark and Delicious Homemade Chili
21. Hungarian Goulash
22. Karen's Hearty Shepherd's Pie
23. Curried Tomato Chicken
24. Honey and Garlic Pork Spareribs
25. Spinach Lasagne

SMOOTHIES

Banana Blueberry Smoothies

(SERVES 2)

Blueberries are high in antioxidants. The combination of two fruits and orange juice makes these smoothies healthy and nutritious.

This was Jeff's favourite smoothie recipe. He really enjoyed his smoothies at breakfast or as an afternoon snack after cancer treatments.

1 small banana, peeled and cut into chunks

½ cup frozen blueberries (antioxidant)

1 cup orange juice with calcium (antioxidant)

2 tablespoons strawberry yogurt, if desired, for a richer taste (antioxidant)

1. Place banana and blueberries in a blender.
2. Pour orange juice into blender.
3. Cover and blend until smooth.

◆ ◆ ◆

Banana Raspberry Smoothies

(SERVES 2)

These smoothies are a great way to start the morning. Raspberries are cancer-preventing berries and these delicious drinks are a real morale booster during cancer treatments and post-treatment recovery.

1 small banana, peeled and cut into chunks

½ cup frozen raspberries (antioxidant)

1 cup orange juice with calcium (antioxidant)

2 tablespoons strawberry yogurt, if desired, for a richer taste (antioxidant)

1. Place banana and raspberries in a blender.
2. Pour orange juice into blender.
3. Cover and blend until smooth.

◆ ◆ ◆

Banana Strawberry Smoothies

(SERVES 2)

Jeff enjoyed these energy booster drinks most in the afternoon after cancer treatments. Strawberries are another anti-cancer fruit.

1 small banana, peeled and cut into chunks

½ cup frozen strawberries (antioxidant)

1 cup orange juice with calcium (antioxidant)

2 tablespoons strawberry yogurt, if desired, for a richer taste (antioxidant)

1. Place banana and raspberries in a blender.
2. Pour orange juice into blender.
3. Cover and blend until smooth.

◆　◆　◆

Citrus Blueberry Smoothies

(SERVES 4)

Blueberries are at the top of the list of antioxidant-rich foods, and this was one of the smoothie recipes Jeff enjoyed most. He enjoyed these energy booster drinks in the afternoon after cancer treatments.

3½ cups crushed ice

⅓ cup frozen pink lemonade (or yellow lemonade)

1¼ cups fresh or frozen blueberries (antioxidant)

¾ cup orange juice with calcium (antioxidant)

1. Pour all ingredients into a blender.
2. Cover and blend until smooth.

◆ ◆ ◆

Strawberry Smoothies

(SERVES 4)

Strawberries are abundant in antioxidants. These smoothies were one of Jeff's favourites, often enjoyed in the afternoon after cancer treatments.

- **3 cups crushed ice**
- **⅓ cup frozen pink lemonade (or limeade)**
- **2 cups strawberries, hulled and halved** (antioxidant)
- **4–5 tablespoons icing sugar**

1. Pour all ingredients into a blender.
2. Cover and blend until smooth.

◆ ◆ ◆

APPETIZERS

Beef and Black Bean Tortilla Chip Dip, 42

Chicken Quesadillas, 43

Guacamole, 44

Hummus Dip, 45

Karen's Crab-Stuffed Mushroom Caps, 46

Karen's Nacho Chips, 47

Tzatziki (Yogurt-Cucumber Dip), 48

Vegetarian Quesadillas, 49

Beef and Black Bean Tortilla Chip Dip
(SERVES 6–8)

This recipe is loaded with antioxidants and powerful anti-cancer nutrients from tomatoes and beans. This was Jeff's favourite dip recipe and an ideal appetizer, afternoon snack or lunch treat.

Keep leftover dip in a covered container in the refrigerator. It can be reheated in the microwave the next day.

1½ lbs lean ground beef

1¼ tablespoons chili powder

1 × 19 oz/540 mL can black beans, drained well (antioxidant)

¾ cup restaurant style chunky salsa

6 medium Roma tomatoes, seeded and diced (antioxidant)

2 green onions, chopped (antioxidant)

¼–⅓ cup sliced ripe black olives, drained well

1 × 14 oz/398 mL can artichoke hearts, drained well and chopped

natural corn tortilla chips

1. Crumble beef in a large saucepan. Stir in chili powder. Cook over medium-high heat until meat is no longer pink inside. Drain fat.
2. Stir in black beans and chunky salsa. Reduce heat to medium-low and cook until heated through.
3. Spread beef mixture evenly in the bottom of a 9-inch pie plate.
4. Top with tomatoes, green onions, olives and artichokes.
5. Serve with tortilla chips.

◆ ◆ ◆

Chicken Quesadillas

(SERVES 4)

This recipe came in handy after Jeff's medical appointments. This is a quick meal for lunch or dinner.

4 medium-size soft flour tortillas

½ cup light Cheddar cheese, shredded

½ cup light mozzarella cheese, shredded (antioxidant) (or Swiss cheese)

4 thinly sliced cooked chicken or turkey breasts

2 green onions, chopped (antioxidant)

2 medium tomatoes, seeded and chopped (antioxidant)

1. Place tortilla in a 7½-inch non-stick skillet.
2. Sprinkle cheeses, then meat, onions and tomatoes over tortilla.
3. Cook over medium heat until cheese melts. Fold tortilla in half. Press firmly with a spatula.
4. Remove to a warm serving platter.
5. Repeat with remaining tortillas and ingredients.
6. Cut each tortilla into three wedges.

◆ ◆ ◆

Guacamole

(MAKES ABOUT 2 CUPS)

This is a quick and healthy dip recipe to make for an appetizer. It is best served on the same day that it is prepared.

> **2 large ripe avocados, pitted, peeled and mashed with a fork** (antioxidant)
> **⅓ cup chunky salsa**
> **1 tablespoon lime juice (or lemon juice)** (antioxidant)
> **tortilla chips**

1. Combine all ingredients, except chips, in a serving bowl until well mixed.
2. Chill in refrigerator before serving with tortilla chips.

◆　◆　◆

Hummus Dip

(MAKES ABOUT 2 CUPS)

This is a healthy appetizer dip to enjoy after cancer treatments.

Leftover dip is best kept in a covered container in the refrigerator and is just as great-tasting the next day.

1 × 19 oz/540 mL can chickpeas, drained well
1½ tablespoons all natural tahini sesame paste
¼ cup extra virgin olive oil (antioxidant)
juice of 1 lemon (antioxidant)
2 cloves garlic, peeled and minced (antioxidant)
salt, to taste
freshly ground black pepper, to taste
pita bread wedges (or substitute carrot and celery sticks)

1. Place all ingredients, except pita bread, in a food processor.
2. Process until mixture is smooth.
3. Serve with pita bread wedges.

◆ ◆ ◆

Karen's Crab-Stuffed Mushroom Caps

(MAKES 16–18 LARGE)

These mushroom caps were Jeff's favourite appetizers. They were a big morale booster for him in the afternoon while he was recovering from cancer treatments.

Leftovers are best kept in a covered container in the refrigerator. They can be reheated in the microwave the following day.

16–18 large white mushroom caps, washed and dried, stems removed and reserved

½ mushroom stems, chopped finely

8 oz/225 g block light cream cheese, softened at room temperature

2–3 stalks green onions, chopped (use green part only) (antioxidant)

1 × 4 oz/120 g can crabmeat, drained well

dash of dry white wine (optional)

1½–2 cups light Swiss cheese, shredded

1½–2 cups light medium Cheddar cheese, shredded

salt, to taste

freshly ground black pepper, to taste

1. Place prepared mushroom caps upside down in a 9×13×2-inch glass baking dish.
2. Combine remaining ingredients in a mixing bowl until well blended.
3. Spoon crabmeat mixture into mushroom caps. Fill to the top.
4. Bake, on middle oven rack, in a preheated 350°F oven for 35 to 45 minutes until fully cooked.

◆ ◆ ◆

Karen's Nacho Chips

(SERVES 6–8)

This recipe is loaded with antioxidants from the tomatoes, avocados and mozzarella cheese. It is an ideal recipe for lunch or brunch. Jeff enjoyed these nachos while he was recovering from cancer treatments.

1 bag of stone-ground yellow corn nacho chips

5–6 medium tomatoes, seeded and chopped (antioxidant)

2–3 medium ripe avocados, pitted, peeled and diced (antioxidant)

1 bunch green onions, chopped (antioxidant)

3–4 medium fresh green jalapeños, seeded and sliced (or ½ jar of pickled sliced jalapeños)

½ × 14 oz/398 mL can sliced ripe black olives, drained well

1 cup chunky salsa

2–2½ cups light mozzarella cheese, grated (antioxidant)

2–2½ cups light medium Cheddar cheese, grated

1. Place half the nacho chips in a single layer in the bottom of a 10-inch or 11-inch round glass baking dish.

2. Top with half the tomatoes first and end with half of the cheeses.

3. Layer with remaining chips.

4. Top with remaining ingredients.

5. Bake, on middle oven rack, in a preheated 350°F oven for 35 to 45 minutes. Broil 5 minutes longer to brown the cheeses.

◆ ◆ ◆

Tzatziki (Yogurt-Cucumber Dip)

(SERVES 4)

This is a light appetizer dip, which goes well with vegetable sticks. This recipe is loaded with antioxidants.

1 long English cucumber, peeled and grated

1¼ cups plain yogurt (antioxidant)

salt, to taste

freshly ground black pepper, to taste

dash of garlic powder

juice of half a lemon (antioxidant)

carrot and celery sticks (antioxidants)

1. Combine all ingredients, except carrots and celery, in a serving bowl until well blended.

2. Refrigerate and serve cold with vegetables.

♦ ♦ ♦

Vegetarian Quesadillas

(SERVES 6)

This is an ideal meatless recipe for a lighter lunch or brunch. These stuffed tortillas can be served for dinner with a tossed green salad.

8 oz/2 cups light Cheddar cheese, shredded

½ cup tomatoes, seeded and chopped (antioxidant)

3 medium green onions, chopped (antioxidant)

6 large-size soft flour tortillas

1. Place 3 tortillas on each large baking sheet.
2. Top with cheese first, then tomatoes, and green onions last on half side of each tortilla. Fold tortilla in half.
3. Bake, on middle oven rack, in a preheated 350°F oven for 5 to 7 minutes until cheese is melted.
4. Cut each tortilla into three triangular wedges with a knife.

◆ ◆ ◆

COOKIES

Chocolate Chunk Cookies

(MAKES 8 LARGE)

These cookies are a real treat when you have a craving for sweets, as long as you are not counting calories.

They stay fresh for several days in an airtight container.

½ cup (¼ lb) margarine, softened at room temperature

½ cup white granulated sugar

⅓ cup golden yellow sugar

1 cup all-purpose flour

3 tablespoons premium cocoa powder

¾ teaspoon baking powder

dash of salt

1 large egg, beaten (antioxidant)

1 teaspoon vanilla extract

100 g milk chocolate bar, cut into small chunks (or premium dark chocolate bar as a substitute)

1 cup all natural shelled walnuts, chopped

1. Cream margarine in a large mixing bowl with a wooden spoon.
2. Add remaining ingredients and mix well.
3. Knead dough by hand and gather into a large ball. Refrigerate dough in a covered bowl for about 45 minutes.
4. Divide dough into eight equal portions. Shape each portion into a ball. Place four cookies on each baking sheet. Press with fingers to flatten slightly.
5. Bake cookies, on upper one-third of oven rack, in a preheated 350°F oven for 18 to 20 minutes.

◆ ◆ ◆

Date Spice Cookies
(MAKES 11 LARGE SIZE)

These cookies are hearty and full of flavour. Jeff found that half a cookie was ideal for restoring his energy level between attending cancer appointments and eating meals at home.

These cookies can be stored in an airtight container for several days.

1 cup (½ lb) margarine, softened at room temperature

1½ cups golden yellow sugar

3 cups all-purpose flour

1¼ teaspoons baking powder

1 teaspoon baking soda

dash of salt

1 tablespoon ground nutmeg

dash of ground allspice

3 large eggs, beaten (antioxidant)

1½ teaspoons vanilla extract

¾ cup sultana raisins

1⅔ cups dates, chopped

¾ cup all natural shelled walnuts, chopped

1. Cream margarine in a large mixing bowl with a wooden spoon.
2. Add remaining ingredients and mix well.
3. Knead dough by hand and gather into a large ball. Divide dough into eleven equal portions. Shape each portion into a ball. Place four cookies on each baking sheet. Press with fingers to flatten slightly.
4. Bake cookies, on upper one-third of oven rack, in a preheated 375°F oven for about 18 minutes.

◆ ◆ ◆

Giant Chocolate Chip Cookies

(MAKES 8 4¾-INCH SIZE)

This recipe is a real success with all ages. These cookies are lighter in texture and not overly sweet.

These cookies can be stored in an airtight container for several days.

- ½ cup (¼ lb) margarine square, softened at room temperature
- 1¼ cups golden yellow sugar
- ½ cup white granulated sugar
- 3 cups all-purpose flour
- 1½ teaspoons baking soda
- ¾ teaspoon salt
- 1 large egg, beaten (antioxidant)
- 1 teaspoon vanilla extract
- ⅓ cup cold water
- 1¾ cups semi-sweet chocolate chips
- ½ cup all natural shelled walnuts, chopped (optional)

1. Cream margarine in a large mixing bowl with a wooden spoon.
2. Add remaining ingredients and mix well.
3. Knead dough by hand and gather into a large ball. Divide into eight equal portions. Shape each portion into a ball. Place four cookies on each baking sheet. Press with fingers to flatten slightly.
4. Bake cookies, on upper one-third of oven rack, in a preheated 325°F oven for 23 to 25 minutes.

◆ ◆ ◆

Giant Chocolate Chip Walnut Cookies
(MAKES 8 LARGE)

This is one of our favourite cookie recipes. Jeff enjoyed half a cookie with a glass of skim milk in the afternoon.

These cookies can be stored in an airtight container for several days.

1 cup (½ lb) margarine, softened at room temperature

¾ cup golden yellow sugar

¾ cup white granulated sugar

2¼ cups all-purpose flour

1 teaspoon baking soda

dash of salt

2 large eggs, beaten (antioxidant)

1 teaspoon vanilla extract

1¾ cups semi-sweet chocolate chips

1½ cups all natural shelled walnuts, chopped

1. Cream margarine in a large mixing bowl with a wooden spoon.
2. Add remaining ingredients and mix well.
3. Knead dough by hand and gather into a large ball. Divide dough into eight equal portions. Shape each portion into a ball. Place four cookies on each baking sheet. Press with fingers to flatten slightly.
4. Bake cookies, on upper one-third of oven rack, in a preheated 350°F oven for about 20 minutes.

◆ ◆ ◆

Giant Coconut Raisin Cranberry Oatmeal Cookies

(MAKES 8 4¾-INCH SIZE)

These cookies are loaded with antioxidants. They are a tasty way to get your oatmeal supplement for the day.

These cookies can be stored in an airtight container for several days.

1 cup (½ lb) margarine, softened at room temperature

2 cups golden yellow sugar

2 cups all-purpose flour

2 cups quick cooking oats (antioxidant)

1 teaspoon baking powder

½ teaspoon baking soda

dash of salt

2 large eggs, beaten (antioxidant)

¾ teaspoon vanilla extract

1½ cups sweetened shredded coconut

¾ cup sultana raisins

½ cup sweetened dried cranberries (antioxidant)

1. Cream margarine in a large mixing bowl with a wooden spoon.

2. Stir in remaining ingredients until well mixed.

3. Knead dough by hand and gather into a large ball. Divide dough into eight equal portions. Shape each portion into a ball. Place four cookies on each baking sheet. Press with fingers to flatten slightly.

4. Bake cookies, on upper one-third of oven rack, in a preheated 350°F oven for 22 to 24 minutes.

◆ ◆ ◆

Giant Double Chocolate Walnut Cookies

(MAKES 10 4-INCH SIZE)

This was Jeff's favourite cookie recipe. I baked these cookies many times and he often enjoyed a whole cookie with a glass of skim milk. The treat always gave him a big morale lift after medical appointments or while he was recuperating from cancer treatments.

These cookies can be stored in an airtight container for several days.

- ½ cup (¼ lb) margarine, softened at room temperature
- 2 cups golden yellow sugar
- 3 cups all-purpose flour
- ½ cup premium cocoa powder
- 1 tablespoon baking soda
- ¼ teaspoon salt
- 3 extra-large eggs, beaten (antioxidant)
- 5 tablespoons corn syrup (or honey)
- ¾ tablespoon vanilla extract
- 1½ cups semi-sweet chocolate chips (or 2½ cups premium dark chocolate bar, cut into small chunks)
- 1½ cups all natural shelled walnuts, chopped

1. Cream margarine in a large mixing bowl with a wooden spoon.
2. Stir in remaining ingredients and mix well. Knead dough by hand and gather into a large ball. Divide dough into ten equal portions. Shape each portion into a ball. Place four cookies on each baking sheet. Press with fingers to flatten slightly.
3. Bake cookies, on upper one-third of oven rack, in a preheated 325°F oven for 20 minutes.

◆ ◆ ◆

Giant Oatmeal Blueberry Cranberry Cookies

(MAKES 12 4½-INCH SIZE)

This is one of our family's most-loved recipes. These cookies are loaded with antioxidants from blueberries and cranberries and a great way to get oatmeal in your diet.

These cookies can be stored in an airtight container for several days.

- 1 cup (½ lb) margarine, softened at room temperature
- 1 cup white granulated sugar
- 1 cup golden yellow sugar
- 2 cups all-purpose flour
- 2 cups quick cooking oats (antioxidant)
- sprinkle of nutmeg
- 1 teaspoon baking powder
- 1 teaspoon baking soda
- ½ teaspoon salt
- 2 extra-large eggs, beaten (antioxidant)
- 1 tablespoon vanilla extract
- ¾ cup sweetened dried blueberries (antioxidant)
- 1¾ cups sweetened dried cranberries (antioxidant)

1. Cream margarine in a large mixing bowl with a wooden spoon.
2. Stir in remaining ingredients and mix well.
3. Knead dough by hand and gather into a large ball. Divide dough into twelve equal portions. Shape each portion into a ball. Place four cookies on each baking sheet. Press with fingers to flatten slightly.
4. Bake cookies, on upper one-third of oven rack, in a preheated 350°F oven for 20 minutes.

◆ ◆ ◆

Giant Oatmeal Chocolate Chip Raisin Cookies

(MAKES 12 4½-INCH SIZE)

These cookies have a soft and chewy texture from the raisins and chocolate chips.

These cookies can be stored in an airtight container for several days.

- 1 cup (½ lb) margarine, softened at room temperature
- 1 cup white granulated sugar
- 1 cup golden yellow sugar
- 2 cups all-purpose flour
- 2 cups quick cooking oats (antioxidant)
- sprinkle of nutmeg
- 1 teaspoon baking powder
- 1 teaspoon baking soda
- ½ teaspoon salt
- 2 extra-large eggs, beaten (antioxidant)
- 1 tablespoon vanilla extract
- 1⅓ cups semi-sweet chocolate chips
- 1⅓ cups sultana raisins

1. Cream margarine in a large mixing bowl with a wooden spoon.
2. Stir in remaining ingredients and mix well.
3. Knead dough by hand and gather into a large ball. Divide dough into twelve equal portions. Shape each portion into a ball. Place four cookies on each baking sheet. Press with fingers to flatten slightly.
4. Bake cookies, on upper one-third of oven rack, in a preheated 350°F oven for 20 minutes.

◆ ◆ ◆

Giant Oatmeal Chocolate Cookies

(MAKES 12 4½-INCH SIZE)

These colourful cookies taste as scrumptious as they appear.

These cookies can be stored in an airtight container for several days.

1 cup (½ lb) margarine, softened at room temperature

1 cup white granulated sugar

1 cup golden yellow sugar

2 cups all-purpose flour

2 cups quick cooking oats (antioxidant)

sprinkle of nutmeg

1 teaspoon baking powder

1 teaspoon baking soda

½ teaspoon salt

2 extra-large eggs, beaten (antioxidant)

1 tablespoon vanilla extract

1⅓ cups candy-coated chocolate pieces

1. Cream margarine in a large mixing bowl with a wooden spoon.
2. Stir in remaining ingredients and mix well.
3. Knead dough by hand and gather into a large ball. Divide dough into twelve equal portions. Shape each portion into a ball. Place four cookies on each baking sheet. Press with fingers to flatten slightly.
4. Bake cookies, on upper one-third of oven rack, in a preheated 350°F oven for 20 minutes.

◆ ◆ ◆

Giant Oatmeal Cranberry Raisin Cookies

(MAKES 12 4½-INCH SIZE)

These delicious cookies are a real success with all ages and one of Jeff's favourite cookies. They are also a healthy alternative to store-bought cookies. These cookies are full of antioxidants. We enjoyed sharing one after medical appointments. They contributed to alleviating constipation when he was taking many prescribed medications during his cancer treatments.

These cookies can be stored in an airtight container for several days.

1 cup (½ lb) margarine, softened at room temperature
1 cup white granulated sugar
1 cup golden yellow sugar
2 cups all-purpose flour
2 cups quick cooking oats (antioxidant)
sprinkle of nutmeg
1 teaspoon baking powder
1 teaspoon baking soda
½ teaspoon salt
2 extra-large eggs, beaten (antioxidant)
1 tablespoon vanilla extract
1⅓ cups sultana raisins
1⅓ cups sweetened dried cranberries (antioxidant)

1. Cream margarine in a large mixing bowl with a wooden spoon.
2. Stir in remaining ingredients and mix well.
3. Knead dough by hand and gather into a large ball. Divide dough into twelve equal portions. Shape each portion into a ball. Place four cookies on each baking sheet. Press with fingers to flatten slightly.
4. Bake cookies, on upper one-third of oven rack, in a preheated 350°F oven for 20 minutes.

◆ ◆ ◆

Hearty Oatmeal Spice Cookies

(MAKES 12 LARGE SIZE)

These nutritious cookies are meant to be shared with a loved one. Jeff really enjoyed these cookies after cancer appointments. Half a cookie is sufficient as a snack.

These cookies can be stored in an airtight container for several days.

1 cup (½ lb) margarine, softened at room temperature

1 cup golden yellow sugar

½ cup white granulated sugar

2½ cups all-purpose flour

2 ⅛ cups quick cooking oats (antioxidant)

1 teaspoon baking soda

generous sprinkle of nutmeg

2 large eggs, beaten (antioxidant)

1½ teaspoons vanilla extract

1½ cups all natural walnuts, chopped

1½ cups dark California raisins

1¼ cups sultana raisins

1. Cream margarine in a large mixing bowl with a wooden spoon.
2. Stir in remaining ingredients and mix well.
3. Knead dough by hand and gather into a large ball. Divide dough into twelve equal portions. Shape each portion into a ball. Place four cookies on each baking sheet. Press with fingers to flatten slightly.
4. Bake cookies, on upper one-third of oven rack, in a preheated 375°F oven for 18 to 19 minutes.

◆ ◆ ◆

Jumbo Cranberry White Chocolate Oatmeal Cookies

(MAKES 6 5¼-INCH SIZE)

These spiced cookies are chewy and full of antioxidants. This is an ideal recipe for those who prefer white chocolate chips to milk chocolate chips.

These cookies can be stored in an airtight container for several days.

1 cup (½ lb) margarine, softened at room temperature

1 cup golden yellow sugar

½ cup white granulated sugar

1½ cups all-purpose flour

2 cups quick cooking oats (antioxidant)

1¼ teaspoons baking powder

½ teaspoon baking soda

dash of salt

1 teaspoon ground nutmeg

dash of ground allspice

dash of ground cloves

2 large eggs, beaten (antioxidant)

¾ teaspoon vanilla extract

¾ cup sweetened dried cranberries (antioxidant)

½ cup white chocolate chips

1. Cream margarine in a large mixing bowl with a wooden spoon.
2. Stir in remaining ingredients and mix well.
3. Knead dough by hand and gather into a large ball. Divide dough into six equal portions. Shape each portion into a ball. Place three cookies on each baking sheet. Press with fingers to flatten slightly.
4. Bake cookies, on upper one-third of oven rack, in a preheated 350°F oven for 22 to 23 minutes.

• • •

Lower-Fat Cranberry Chocolate Oatmeal Cookies

(MAKES 6 4 ¼ TO 4 ½-INCH SIZE)

These colourful cookies make a sweet snack, if you don't mind the extra calories.

These cookies can be stored in an airtight container for several days.

2 tablespoons margarine, softened at room temperature

1 ¾ cups golden yellow sugar

1 ½ cups all-purpose flour

1 cup quick cooking oats (antioxidant)

1 teaspoon baking soda

sprinkle of nutmeg

dash of salt

1 large egg, beaten (antioxidant)

1 large egg white, beaten

¾ tablespoon vanilla extract

¾ cup sweetened dried cranberries (antioxidant)

¾ cup candy-coated chocolate pieces

1. Cream margarine in a large mixing bowl with a wooden spoon.
2. Stir in remaining ingredients and mix well.
3. Knead dough by hand and gather into a large ball. Divide dough into six equal portions. Shape each portion into a ball. Place three cookies on each baking sheet. Press with fingers to flatten slightly.
4. Bake cookies, on upper one-third of oven rack, in a preheated 300°F oven for 22 minutes.

◆ ◆ ◆

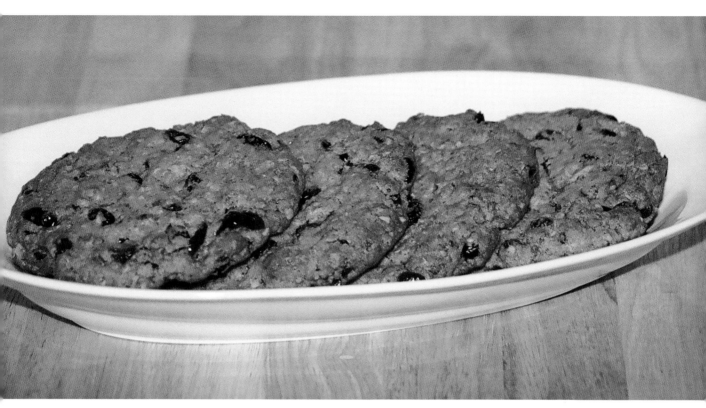

Giant Oatmeal Cranberry Raisin Cookies
Recipe on Page 61

Giant Double Chocolate Walnut Cookies
Recipe on Page 57

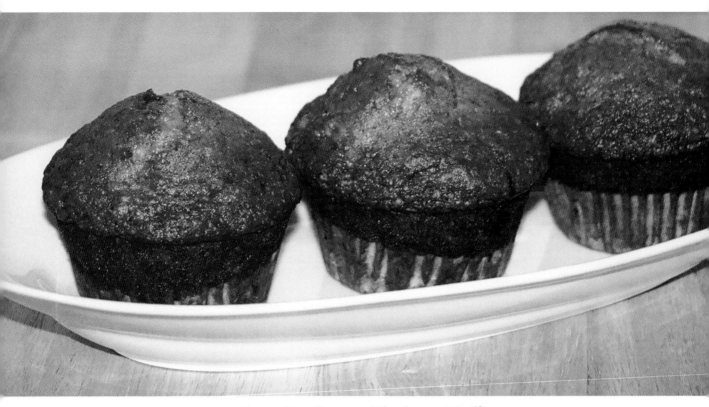

Texas-Size Banana Blueberry Muffins
Recipe on Page 85

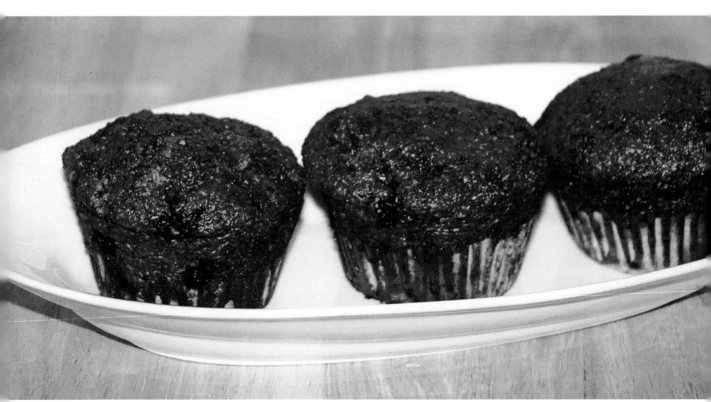

Large Blueberry Bran Muffins
Recipe on Page 81

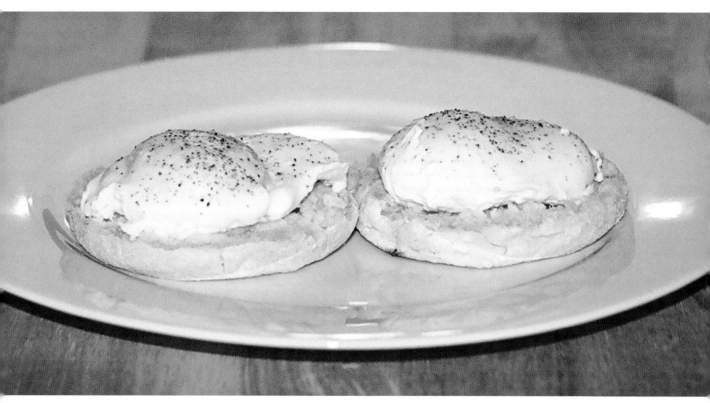

Poached Eggs on English Muffins
Recipe on Page 110

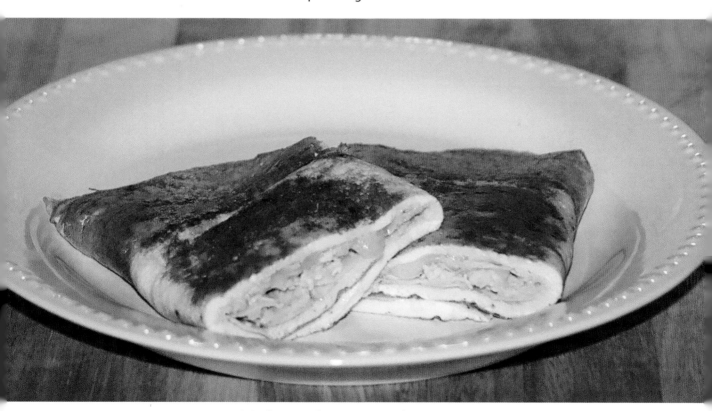

Turkey and Swiss Omelette
Recipe on Page 112

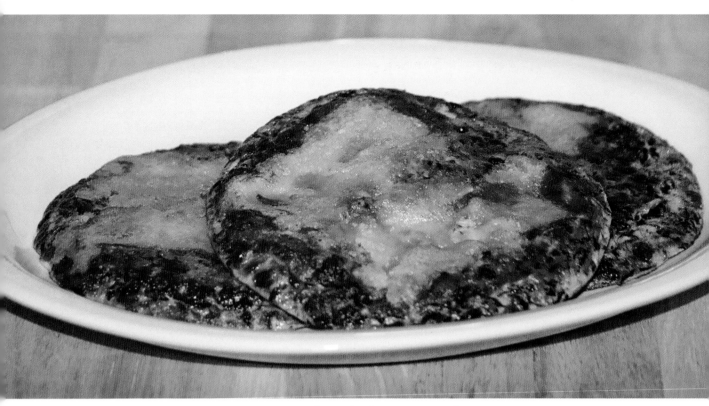

Spinach and Cheese Pancakes
Recipe on Page 114

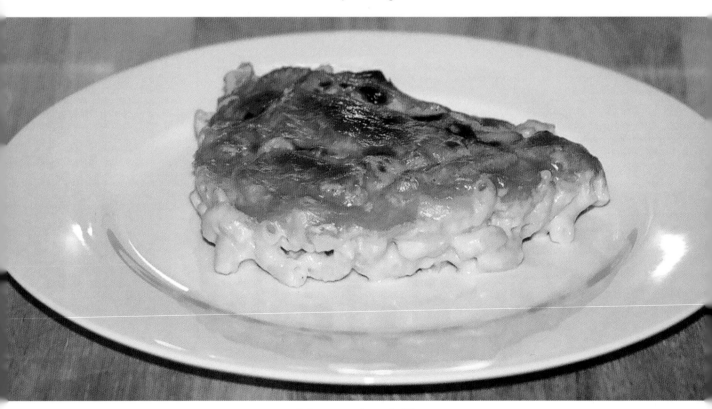

Macaroni and Cheese
Recipe on Page 211

Lower-Fat Oatmeal Raisin Cookies

(MAKES 6 4 ¼ TO 4 ½-INCH SIZE)

These healthy and nutritious cookies are low in both fat and calories. They taste delicious, too.

Half a cookie was ideal as a snack for Jeff during his cancer treatments, especially when weight gain was unavoidable due to taking prescribed medications and reduced physical activities.

These cookies can be stored in an airtight container for several days.

2 tablespoons margarine, softened at room temperature

1 ¾ cups golden yellow sugar

1 ½ cups all-purpose flour

1 cup quick cooking oats (antioxidant)

1 teaspoon baking soda

sprinkle of nutmeg

dash of salt

1 large egg, beaten (antioxidant)

1 large egg white, beaten

¾ tablespoon vanilla extract

1 ½ cups sultana raisins

1. Cream margarine in a large mixing bowl with a wooden spoon.
2. Stir in remaining ingredients and mix well.
3. Knead dough by hand and gather into a large ball. Divide dough into six equal portions. Shape each portion into a ball. Place three cookies on each baking sheet. Press with fingers to flatten slightly.
4. Bake cookies, on upper one-third of oven rack, in a preheated 300°F oven for 22 minutes.

◆ ◆ ◆

Lower-Fat Triple Fruit Oatmeal Cookies

(MAKES 6 4¼ TO 4½-INCH SIZE)

These cookies are low in both fat and calories.

Half a cookie was an ideal snack for Jeff during his cancer treatments, especially when weight gain was unavoidable due to taking prescribed medications and reduced physical activities.

These cookies are best stored in an airtight container for several days.

2 tablespoons margarine, softened at room temperature

1¾ cups golden yellow sugar

1½ cups all-purpose flour

1 cup quick cooking oats (antioxidant)

1 teaspoon baking soda

sprinkle of nutmeg

dash of salt

1 large egg, beaten (antioxidant)

1 large egg white, beaten

¾ tablespoon vanilla extract

½ cup dark California raisins

½ cup dried apricots, chopped (antioxidant)

½ cup dried mangoes, chopped (antioxidant)

1. Cream margarine in a large mixing bowl with a wooden spoon.
2. Stir in remaining ingredients and mix well.
3. Knead dough by hand and gather into a large ball. Divide dough into six equal portions. Shape each portion into a ball. Place three cookies on each baking sheet. Press with fingers to flatten slightly.
4. Bake cookies, on upper one-third of oven rack, in a preheated 300°F oven for 22 minutes.

◆ ◆ ◆

Monster-Size Chocolate Chip Raisin Walnut Cookies
(MAKES 6 EXTRA-LARGE)

These cookies are sweet and crunchy. Half a cookie is sufficient as a snack.

These cookies can be stored in an airtight container for several days.

1 cup (½ lb) margarine, softened at room temperature

1¼ cups golden yellow sugar

2 cups all-purpose flour

1½ teaspoons baking soda

dash of salt, to taste

1 large egg, beaten (antioxidant)

1 teaspoon vanilla extract

1½ cups semi-sweet chocolate chips

½ cup sultana raisins (or sweetened dried cranberries)

1½ cups all natural shelled walnuts, chopped

1. Cream margarine in a large mixing bowl with a wooden spoon.
2. Add remaining ingredients and mix well.
3. Knead dough by hand and gather into a large ball. Divide dough into six equal portions. Shape each portion into a ball. Place three cookies on each baking sheet. Press with fingers to flatten slightly.
4. Bake cookies, on upper one-third of oven rack, in a preheated 350°F oven for about 20 minutes.

◆ ◆ ◆

The Very Best Chunky Peanut Butter Cookies

(MAKES 14 3 ¾ TO 4-INCH SIZE)

You will not find a cookie recipe like this one. These cookies smell and taste wonderful. This was one of Jeff's favourite cookies for after cancer treatments or when weight gain was necessary.

These cookies can be stored in an airtight container for several days.

1 cup (½ lb) margarine, softened at room temperature

1 cup white granulated sugar

1 cup golden yellow sugar

3 cups all-purpose flour

1 teaspoon salt

1 teaspoon baking soda

2 cups crunchy peanut butter (light preferred)

2 extra-large eggs, beaten (antioxidant)

1 teaspoon vanilla extract

3 cups natural walnuts, chopped

1. Cream margarine in a large mixing bowl with a wooden spoon.
2. Add remaining ingredients and mix well.
3. Knead dough by hand and gather into a large ball. Divide dough into fourteen equal portions. Shape each portion into a ball. Place four cookies on each baking sheet. Press with fingers to flatten slightly.
4. Bake cookies, on upper one-third of oven rack, in a preheated 325°F oven for 30 minutes.

◆ ◆ ◆

The Very Best Peanut Butter Chocolate Chunk Cookies

(MAKES 14 3¾ TO 4-INCH SIZE)

These cookies are decadent and not low in calories. They are ideal for times when weight loss occurs.

These cookies can be stored in an airtight container for several days.

- 1 cup (½ lb) margarine, softened at room temperature
- 1 cup white granulated sugar
- 1 cup golden yellow sugar
- 3 cups all-purpose flour
- 1 teaspoon salt
- 1 teaspoon baking soda
- 2 cups crunchy peanut butter (light preferred)
- 2 extra-large eggs, beaten (antioxidant)
- 1 teaspoon vanilla extract
- 1 cup natural walnuts, chopped
- 1 cup premium Swiss chocolate bar, cut into small chunks

1. Cream margarine in a large mixing bowl with a wooden spoon.
2. Add remaining ingredients and mix well.
3. Knead dough by hand and gather into a large ball. Divide dough into fourteen equal portions. Shape each portion into a ball. Place four cookies on each baking sheet. Press with fingers to flatten slightly.
4. Bake cookies, on upper one-third of oven rack, in a preheated 325°F oven for 30 minutes.

◆ ◆ ◆

MUFFINS

Banana Coconut Muffins

(MAKES 9 LARGE SIZE)

This is a great muffin recipe, especially if you enjoy the taste of bananas and coconut together.

These muffins can be stored in an airtight container for 2 to 3 days. They freeze well in freezer bags for up to 3 months.

7 large very ripe bananas, peeled and mashed

1½ cups white granulated sugar

2 large eggs, beaten (antioxidant)

5 tablespoons canola oil

3 cups all-purpose flour

1 tablespoon baking powder

1 tablespoon baking soda

1 teaspoon salt

1 cup sweetened shredded coconut

1. Combine bananas, sugar, eggs and oil in a large mixing bowl.
2. Stir in remaining ingredients until just mixed.
3. Spoon batter into paper-lined 3½-inch size muffin cups.
4. Bake muffins, on middle oven rack, in a preheated 375°F oven for 20 minutes. Then lower oven temperature to 325°F and bake another 10 to 15 minutes more.

◆ ◆ ◆

Banana Cranberry Muffins

(MAKES 9 LARGE SIZE)

These low-fat muffins have the great flavours of bananas and cranberries.

These muffins can be stored in an airtight container for 2 to 3 days. They freeze well in freezer bags for up to 3 months.

7 large very ripe bananas, peeled and mashed

1½ cups white granulated sugar

2 large eggs, beaten (antioxidant)

5 tablespoons canola oil

3 cups all-purpose flour

1 tablespoon baking powder

1 tablespoon baking soda

1 teaspoon salt

1 cup sweetened dried cranberries (or frozen cranberries) (antioxidant)

1. Combine bananas, sugar, eggs and oil in a large mixing bowl.
2. Stir in remaining ingredients until just mixed.
3. Spoon batter into paper-lined 3½-inch size muffin cups.
4. Bake muffins, on middle oven rack, in a preheated 375°F oven for 20 minutes. Then reduce oven temperature to 325°F and bake another 10 to 15 minutes more.

◆ ◆ ◆

Big Coconut Raisin Muffins

(MAKES 10 LARGE SIZE)

This recipe has been popular with everyone. These muffins are moist and not overly sweet.

These muffins can be stored in an airtight container for 2 to 3 days. They freeze well in freezer bags for up to 3 months.

3½ cups all-purpose flour

1 cup white granulated sugar

2 cups sweetened shredded coconut

2 tablespoons baking powder

¾ teaspoon salt

1 cup sultana raisins

2 large eggs, beaten (antioxidant)

2 cups skim milk (antioxidant)

½ cup canola oil

candied cherries for decoration, if desired

1. Combine the first six ingredients in a large mixing bowl.
2. Stir in remaining ingredients until well mixed.
3. Spoon batter into paper-lined 3½-inch size muffin cups. Fill each muffin cup almost full.
4. Top each muffin with a cherry, if desired.
5. Bake muffins, on middle oven rack, in a preheated 375°F oven for 20 minutes. Then reduce oven temperature to 325°F and bake another 5 to 8 minutes until done.

◆ ◆ ◆

Carrot Raisin Walnut Muffins

(MAKES 9 LARGE SIZE)

These muffins are hearty and filling and a tasty way to get your carrot supplement in the morning or afternoon.

These muffins can be stored in an airtight container for 2 to 3 days. They freeze well in freezer bags for up to 3 months.

2 cups all-purpose flour

1⅛ cups white granulated sugar

1 tablespoon baking soda

sprinkle of nutmeg

dash of salt

1 cup sultana raisins

¾ cup natural walnuts, chopped

½ cup sweetened shredded coconut

3 large eggs, beaten (antioxidant)

¾ cup canola oil

1 teaspoon vanilla extract

2¼ cups carrots, grated (antioxidant)

1. Combine the first eight ingredients in a large mixing bowl.
2. Add remaining ingredients and stir until just moistened.
3. Spoon batter into paper-lined 3½-inch size muffin cups.
4. Bake muffins, on middle oven rack, in a preheated 325°F oven for 35 to 38 minutes.

◆ ◆ ◆

Chocolate Chip Walnut Surprise Muffins

(MAKES 6 LARGE SIZE)

This is an ideal recipe for when you crave something sweet and you do not want to spend too much time baking. These muffins are not low in calories.

These muffins can be stored in an airtight container for 2 to 3 days. They freeze well in freezer bags for up to 3 months.

> 2 cups all-purpose flour
> ¾ cup white granulated sugar
> 1 tablespoon baking powder
> sprinkle of nutmeg
> ¼ teaspoon baking soda
> dash of salt
> ⅔ cup semi-sweet chocolate chips
> ½ cup natural walnuts, chopped
> 1 large egg, beaten (antioxidant)
> 1 teaspoon vanilla extract
> 1 cup skim milk (antioxidant)
> ½ cup margarine, melted
> 6 tablespoons raspberry jam
> ⅓ cup semi-sweet chocolate chips, extra

1. Combine the first eight ingredients in a large mixing bowl.
2. Add egg, vanilla, milk and margarine. Stir until just moistened.
3. Fill each paper-lined 3½-inch size muffin cup half full of batter. Place 1 tablespoon of jam in centre of batter. Spoon the remaining batter over jam in each muffin cup.
4. Sprinkle remaining chocolate chips evenly over batter in each muffin cup.
5. Bake muffins, on middle oven rack, in a preheated 375°F oven for 25 minutes.

◆ ◆ ◆

Cranberry Apple Walnut Spice Muffins

(MAKES 9 LARGE SIZE)

The combination of nutmeg, applesauce and cranberries makes these muffins very tasty.

These muffins can be stored in an airtight container for 2 to 3 days. They freeze well in freezer bags for up to 3 months.

4 cups all-purpose flour
1 cup white granulated sugar
1 tablespoon baking soda
sprinkle of nutmeg
1 teaspoon salt
1¾ cups unsweetened applesauce
⅛ cup water
⅔ cup canola oil
3 large eggs, beaten (antioxidant)
2 cups frozen cranberries (antioxidant)
1 cup natural walnuts, chopped

1. Combine flour, sugar, soda, nutmeg and salt in a large mixing bowl.
2. Add remaining ingredients and stir until just moistened.
3. Spoon batter into paper-lined 3½-inch muffin cups. Fill each muffin cup almost full.
4. Bake muffins, on middle oven rack, in a preheated 325°F oven for about 40 minutes.

◆ ◆ ◆

Crunchy Peanut Butter Surprise Muffins

(MAKES 9 LARGE SIZE)

Peanut butter and jam go well together in this muffin recipe.

These muffins can be stored in an airtight container for 2 to 3 days. They freeze well in freezer bags for up to 3 months.

> 3 cups all-purpose flour
> 1 cup white granulated sugar
> 2 tablespoons baking powder
> 1 teaspoon salt
> 4 large eggs, beaten (antioxidant)
> 2 cups skim milk (antioxidant)
> 3 tablespoons canola oil
> 1 cup crunchy peanut butter
> 9 teaspoons raspberry jam
> semi-sweet chocolate chips for sprinkling on top

1. Combine flour, sugar, baking powder and salt in a large mixing bowl.
2. Add eggs, milk, oil and peanut butter. Stir until just moistened.
3. Spoon batter into paper-lined 3½-inch muffin cups. Fill each muffin cup half full.
4. Place 1 teaspoon of jam in centre of batter. Fill each muffin cup with remaining batter almost full.
5. Sprinkle chocolate chips on top of batter.
6. Bake muffins, on middle oven rack, in a preheated 375°F oven for 20 minutes. Then lower oven temperature to 325°F and bake another 15 minutes.

◆ ◆ ◆

Extra-Large Triple Berry Muffins
(MAKES 14 LARGE SIZE)

These muffins are loaded with antioxidants from the berries. Half a muffin is sufficient as a snack unless you have a bigger appetite.

These muffins can be stored in an airtight container for 2 to 3 days. They freeze well in freezer bags for up to 3 months.

> 6 cups all-purpose flour
>
> 2¼ cups white granulated sugar
>
> 4 tablespoons baking powder
>
> 1½ teaspoons salt
>
> 6 large eggs, beaten (antioxidant)
>
> 2¼ cups skim milk (antioxidant)
>
> 1½ cups margarine, melted
>
> 3 cups frozen mixed berries (blackberries, blueberries and raspberries) (antioxidants)

1. Combine flour, sugar, baking powder and salt in a large mixing bowl.
2. Add remaining ingredients and stir until just moistened.
3. Spoon batter into paper-lined 3½-inch muffin cups. Fill each muffin cup almost full.
4. Bake muffins, on middle oven rack, in a preheated 350°F oven for 40 to 45 minutes until golden at edges.

◆ ◆ ◆

Giant Blueberry Muffins

(MAKES 12 EXTRA-LARGE SIZE)

These huge muffins are light in texture and fun to share with a loved one. They are a great way to get blueberries in your diet.

These muffins can be stored in an airtight container for 2 to 3 days. They freeze well in freezer bags for up to 3 months.

4 cups all-purpose flour

1½ cups white granulated sugar

2½ tablespoons baking powder

1 teaspoon salt

4 large eggs, beaten (antioxidant)

1½ cups skim milk (antioxidant)

¾ cup margarine, melted and slightly cooled

2½ cups frozen blueberries, partially thawed (antioxidant)

1. Combine flour, sugar, baking powder and salt in a large mixing bowl.
2. Stir in remaining ingredients until well mixed.
3. Spoon batter into paper-lined 3½-inch size muffin cups. Fill each cup almost full.
4. Bake muffins, on middle oven rack, in a preheated 350°F oven for 40 to 45 minutes until golden.

◆ ◆ ◆

Large Blueberry Bran Muffins
(MAKES 6 LARGE SIZE)

This was Jeff's favourite muffin recipe and the best bran muffins you will ever taste. They are very moist and full of antioxidants. In addition, these low-fat muffins contributed to alleviating constipation during cancer treatments due to increased prescribed medications and reduced physical activities.

These muffins can be stored in an airtight container for 2 to 3 days. They freeze well in freezer bags for up to 3 months.

1 cup all-purpose flour

1½ cups 100% natural wheat bran flakes

1 teaspoon baking soda

¾ teaspoon baking powder

¼ teaspoon salt

1 cup dark brown sugar

1 large egg, beaten (antioxidant)

1 cup skim milk (antioxidant) mixed with 1 tablespoon white vinegar, let stand 5 minutes at room temperature

1 tablespoon canola oil

3 tablespoons dark molasses

2¼ cups frozen blueberries (antioxidant) (or substitute mixed berries, such as blackberries, blueberries and raspberries)

1. Combine the first six dry ingredients in a large mixing bowl.
2. Add remaining ingredients and stir until just moistened.
3. Spoon batter into paper-lined 3½-inch size muffin cups.
4. Bake muffins, on middle oven rack, in a preheated 375°F oven for about 27 minutes.

◆ ◆ ◆

Mixed Berry Healthy Muffins
(MAKES 9 LARGE SIZE)

These low-fat muffins are loaded with antioxidants and a great way to get oats, wheat bran and berries into your morning meal.

These muffins can be stored in an airtight container for 2 to 3 days. They freeze well in freezer bags for up to 3 months.

1¼ cups all-purpose flour

1¼ cups quick cooking oats (antioxidant)

1⅓ cups 100% natural wheat bran flakes

⅔ cup golden yellow sugar

1¾ tablespoons baking powder

1 teaspoon baking soda

¾ teaspoon salt

sprinkle of nutmeg

2 large eggs, beaten (antioxidant)

1¾ cups skim milk (antioxidant) mixed with 2 tablespoons white vinegar, let stand 5 minutes at room temperature

⅓ cup canola oil

1 teaspoon vanilla extract

1¾ cups frozen mixed berries (blackberries, blueberries and raspberries) (antioxidants)

1. Combine the first eight dry ingredients in a large mixing bowl.

2. Add remaining ingredients and stir until just moistened. Do not over beat.

3. Spoon batter into paper-lined 3½-inch size muffin cups. Fill each muffin cup ¾ full.

4. Bake muffins, on middle oven rack, in a preheated 400°F oven about 23 minutes.

◆ ◆ ◆

Monster-Size Banana Raisin Bran Muffins

(MAKES 8 LARGE SIZE)

These lower-fat muffins are ideal for breakfast — half a muffin is a great way to start your day. This recipe is also a good way to use overripe bananas.

These muffins can be stored in an airtight container for 2 to 3 days. They freeze well in freezer bags for up to 3 months.

⅓ cup margarine, softened at room temperature

½ cup golden yellow sugar

4½ medium very ripe bananas, peeled and mashed

¼ cup skim milk (antioxidant)

1 teaspoon vanilla extract

2 large eggs, beaten (antioxidant)

1½ cups all-purpose flour

½ cup natural bran (or natural wheat germ (antioxidant))

1 teaspoon baking powder

1 teaspoon baking soda

dash of salt

½ cup sultana raisins

½ cup natural walnuts, chopped

1. Cream margarine in a large mixing bowl with a wooden spoon.
2. Add sugar, bananas, milk, vanilla and eggs. Blend well.
3. Stir in remaining ingredients until just moistened.
4. Spoon batter into paper-lined 3½-inch size muffin cups. Fill cups ¾ full.
5. Bake muffins, on middle oven rack, in a preheated 375°F oven for 20 to 25 minutes.

◆ ◆ ◆

Super Double Chocolate Walnut Muffins

(MAKES 6 LARGE SIZE)

These muffins are a delicious afternoon treat for chocolate fans who do not mind the extra calories. The walnuts in this recipe give it an added crunch.

These muffins can be stored in an airtight container for 2 to 3 days. They freeze well in freezer bags for up to 3 months.

½ cup (¼ lb) margarine

3 × 1 oz/28 g squares semi-sweet chocolate

1 cup skim milk (antioxidant) mixed with 1 tablespoon white vinegar,
   let stand 5 minutes at room temperature

1 large egg, beaten (antioxidant)

1½ teaspoons vanilla extract

2 cups all-purpose flour

1 cup white granulated sugar

1 teaspoon baking soda

¾ cup semi-sweet chocolate chips

½ cup natural walnuts, chopped

1. Melt margarine with chocolate squares in microwave oven, on high heat, for 1½ minutes. Pour mixture into a large mixing bowl.

2. Add remaining ingredients and mix well.

3. Spoon batter into paper-lined 3½-inch muffin cups. Fill each muffin cup almost full.

4. Bake muffins, on middle oven rack, in a preheated 375°F oven for 20 minutes. Then reduce oven temperature to 325°F and bake another 15 minutes.

◆ ◆ ◆

Texas-Size Banana Blueberry Muffins
(MAKES 9 LARGE SIZE)

This is the ultimate banana muffin recipe. These muffins are low in fat and calories, and they are ideal as a snack.

It was a great way to get bananas and blueberries into Jeff's diet regularly.

These muffins can be stored in an airtight container for 2 to 3 days. They freeze well in freezer bags for up to 3 months.

6 large very ripe bananas, peeled and mashed with a potato masher

1½ cups white granulated sugar

2 large eggs, beaten (antioxidant)

4 tablespoons canola oil

3 cups all-purpose flour

1 tablespoon baking powder

1 tablespoon baking soda

1 teaspoon salt

1 cup frozen blueberries (antioxidant)

1. Combine mashed bananas, sugar, eggs and oil in a large mixing bowl.
2. Stir in remaining ingredients until just mixed.
3. Spoon batter into paper-lined 3½-inch size muffin cups.
4. Bake muffins, on middle oven rack, in a preheated 375°F oven for 20 minutes. Then lower oven temperature to 325°F and bake another 10 to 15 minutes until done.

◆ ◆ ◆

Texas-Size Banana Mixed Berry Muffins

(MAKES 9 LARGE SIZE)

This is one of the best muffins you will ever taste. The four fruits used in this recipe make these muffins delicious.

These muffins can be stored in an airtight container for 2 to 3 days. They freeze well in freezer bags for up to 3 months.

> 6 large very ripe bananas, peeled and mashed with a potato masher
>
> 1½ cups white granulated sugar
>
> 2 large eggs, beaten (antioxidant)
>
> 4 tablespoons canola oil
>
> 3 cups all-purpose flour
>
> 1 tablespoon baking powder
>
> 1 tablespoon baking soda
>
> 1 teaspoon salt
>
> 1 cup frozen mixed berries (blackberries, blueberries and raspberries)
> (antioxidants)

1. Combine mashed bananas, sugar, eggs and oil in a large mixing bowl.
2. Stir in remaining ingredients until just mixed.
3. Spoon batter into paper-lined 3½-inch size muffin cups.
4. Bake muffins, on middle oven rack, in a preheated 375°F oven for 20 minutes. Then lower oven temperature to 325°F and bake another 10 to 15 minutes until done.

◆ ◆ ◆

BROWNIES, CAKES, PIES & FRUIT DESSERTS

Chocolate Walnut Brownies

(MAKES 16 LARGE SQUARES)

These brownies are delicious as an afternoon treat. The cocoa and walnuts go well together in this recipe.

These brownies can be stored in an airtight container for several days.

½ cup margarine, melted

2½ cups white granulated sugar

4 large eggs, beaten (antioxidant)

¾ tablespoon vanilla extract

2 cups all-purpose flour

1 cup premium cocoa powder

½ teaspoon baking powder

dash of salt

1 cup natural walnuts, chopped

1. Combine all ingredients in a large mixing bowl. Mix well.
2. Pour batter into a 9×13-inch baking pan.
3. Bake, on middle oven rack, in a preheated 325°F oven for 30 to 35 minutes.
4. Cool before cutting into 16 large squares.

◆　◆　◆

Dark and Rich Brownies

(MAKES 16 LARGE SQUARES)

This is the ultimate brownie recipe for chocolate fans. These are the most decadent brownies you will ever taste; they will disappear very quickly.

These brownies can be stored in an airtight container for several days, if there are any leftovers.

½ cup margarine

2 × 1 oz/28 g squares semi-sweet chocolate

1⅓ cups premium cocoa powder

3 cups white granulated sugar

5 large eggs, beaten (antioxidant)

¾ tablespoon vanilla extract

2 cups all-purpose flour

1 teaspoon baking powder

dash of salt

1¼ cups natural walnuts, chopped

1. Melt margarine and chocolate squares in microwave oven, over high heat, for 1½ minutes. Pour into a large mixing bowl.
2. Stir in cocoa and sugar until well combined.
3. Add remaining ingredients and stir until well blended.
4. Pour batter into a 9×13-inch baking pan.
5. Bake, on middle oven rack, in a preheated 325°F oven for 30 to 35 minutes.

◆ ◆ ◆

Easy-To-Make Chocolate Cake

(MAKES 1 LARGE SIZE)

This quick and easy cake recipe has been a family favourite over the years. It contains no dairy or eggs, so it is a perfect recipe for those with food allergies.

You can bake this cake in advance. It keeps well wrapped in plastic or stored in a large airtight container.

3 cups all-purpose flour

2 cups white granulated sugar

6 tablespoons premium cocoa powder

1 tablespoon baking soda

1 teaspoon salt

2 cups cold water

⅓ cup canola oil

2 tablespoons white vinegar

candy-coated chocolate pieces for decorating

1. Combine the first five ingredients in a large mixing bowl.
2. Stir in remaining ingredients until well mixed.
3. Pour batter into a 9×13-inch baking pan.
4. Bake cake, on middle oven rack, in a preheated 350°F oven for about 35 minutes.
5. Cool at room temperature.
6. Decorate with coloured candies on top.

◆ ◆ ◆

The Very Best Blueberry Crumb Cake

(MAKES 1 LARGE SIZE)

This light cake is loaded with antioxidants, in addition to being the best crumb cake you will ever taste. The sugary topping gives it an added crunch. This was Jeff's favourite cake recipe. He often enjoyed a piece in the afternoon.

Leftover cake is best stored in an airtight container for a few days, if it lasts that long.

CRUMB CAKE:

⅔ cup margarine, softened at room temperature

3 cups all-purpose flour

1 cup white granulated sugar

1½ tablespoons baking powder

1 teaspoon salt

2 large eggs, beaten (antioxidant)

1 teaspoon vanilla extract

1 cup skim milk (antioxidant)

3½ cups frozen blueberries (or substitute mixed berries, such as blackberries, blueberries and raspberries) (antioxidants)

TOPPING:

½ cup all-purpose flour

⅔ cup white granulated sugar

4 tablespoons margarine

1. Cream margarine in a large mixing bowl with a wooden spoon.
2. Stir in 3 cups flour, 1 cup sugar, baking powder and salt.
3. Add eggs, vanilla, milk and berries. Mix well.
4. Pour batter into a 9×13-inch baking pan.
5. For the topping, combine ½ cup flour and ⅔ cup sugar in a small bowl. Cut in 4 tablespoons margarine with a pastry cutter until mixture is crumbly.
6. Sprinkle crumb mixture over cake batter.
7. Bake, on middle oven rack, in a preheated 375°F oven for 40 minutes.

◆ ◆ ◆

The Very Best Dark Chocolate Cake

(MAKES 1 LARGE SIZE)

This dark moist cake is heavenly, a perfect recipe for those who enjoy chocolate and do not mind the extra calories.

Leftover cake is best stored in a covered container in the refrigerator.

CAKE:

1 cup margarine, softened at room temperature

2½ cups white granulated sugar

4 large eggs, beaten (antioxidant)

1 tablespoon vanilla extract

1 cup premium cocoa powder

2 cups hot water

3 cups all-purpose flour

1 tablespoon baking powder

1 tablespoon baking soda

1 teaspoon salt

1. Cream margarine with sugar in a large mixing bowl with a wooden spoon.
2. Stir in eggs and vanilla until well mixed.
3. Dissolve cocoa in hot water in a separate bowl. Add to above mixture.
4. Add remaining ingredients and mix well.
5. Pour batter into two 8-inch or 9-inch round baking pans.
6. Bake, on middle oven rack, in a preheated 350°F oven for 50 to 60 minutes until an inserted wooden toothpick near the centre of the cake comes out clean.
7. Let cool in pans before icing.

ICING:

2½ cups icing sugar

½ cup premium cocoa powder

6 tablespoons margarine, softened at room temperature

¼ cup skim milk (antioxidant) **(or water)**

dash of vanilla extract

candy-coated chocolate pieces for decorating (or substitute sugared fruit slices)

1. Mix all ingredients together in a bowl.
2. Add more milk, if necessary, to reach spreading consistency.
3. Spread icing over tops and sides of cake with a knife.
4. Decorate with coloured candies.

◆ ◆ ◆

9-Inch Apple Pie

(SERVES 8)

This has been a family-favourite recipe over the years. You will be tempted to have a second slice of this homemade apple pie, as long as you don't mind the extra calories.

Leftover pie should be wrapped in plastic and kept chilled in the refrigerator.

DOUBLE CRUST PASTRY:

⅔ cup lard (or substitute ⅔ cup + 2 tablespoons shortening)

2 cups all-purpose flour

¾ teaspoon salt

4–5 tablespoons cold water

1. Combine flour and salt in a mixing bowl.
2. Cut in lard with a pastry cutter until mixture is crumbly.
3. Add water and mix well.
4. Knead dough by hand and gather into a large ball. Divide dough in half. Shape each half into a flattened round. Roll out pastry 1½ inches larger than inverted 9-inch pie plate with a floured rolling pin. Fold pastry in half and place in pie plate. Unfold pastry and pat against bottom and side of pie plate. Trim excess pastry with a knife.

FILLING:

6 cups tart apples, peeled, cored and thinly sliced

1 cup white granulated sugar

2½ tablespoons all-purpose flour

sprinkle of nutmeg

1 teaspoon margarine, cut into cubes

white granulated sugar, extra for sprinkling on top

1. Combine apples, sugar, flour and nutmeg in a large mixing bowl until fruit is well coated.
2. Spoon fruit mixture into pastry-lined 9-inch pie plate.

3. Spread margarine cubes over pie.

4. Place the other pastry crust on top. Trim excess pastry with a knife. Seal and flute edge with tines of fork. Cut four slits on top of crust with a knife.

5. Sprinkle extra sugar on top of crust.

6. Cover edge of pie with aluminum foil. Place pie on a large baking sheet.

7. Bake pie, on lower one-third of oven rack, in a preheated 375°F oven for 25 minutes. Then remove foil and bake another 23 minutes. Broil 5 minutes more to brown the top of the pie.

◆ ◆ ◆

10-Inch Apple Pie

(SERVES 8–10)

This pie is definitely worth the effort, even with the extra calories. The smell of hot apples and spice will bring back memories of a cozy kitchen.

Leftover pie should be wrapped in plastic and kept chilled in the refrigerator.

DOUBLE CRUST PASTRY:

¾ cup + 2 tablespoons lard (or substitute 1 cup shortening)

2⅔ cups all-purpose flour

¾ teaspoon salt

8–9 tablespoons cold water

1. Combine flour and salt in a mixing bowl.
2. Cut in lard with a pastry cutter until mixture is crumbly.
3. Add water and mix well.
4. Knead dough by hand and gather into a large ball. Divide dough in half. Shape each half into a flattened round. Roll out pastry 1½ inches larger than inverted 10-inch pie plate with a floured rolling pin. Fold pastry in half and place in pie plate. Unfold pastry and pat against bottom and side of pie plate. Trim excess pastry with a knife.

FILLING:

9 cups Golden Delicious apples (9–10 medium size), peeled, cored and thinly sliced

1¼ cups white granulated sugar

4 tablespoons all-purpose flour

sprinkle of nutmeg

1½ teaspoons margarine, cut into cubes

white granulated sugar, extra for sprinkling on top

1. Combine apples, sugar, flour and nutmeg in a large mixing bowl until fruit is well coated.
2. Spoon fruit mixture into pastry-lined 10-inch pie plate.

3. Spread margarine cubes over pie.

4. Place the other pastry crust on top. Trim excess pastry with a knife. Seal and flute edge with tines of fork. Cut four slits on top of crust with a knife.

5. Sprinkle extra sugar on top of crust.

6. Cover edge of pie with aluminum foil. Place pie on a large baking sheet.

7. Bake pie, on lower one-third of oven rack, in a preheated 375°F oven for 25 minutes. Then remove foil and bake another 23 minutes. Broil 5 minutes more to brown the top of the pie.

◆ ◆ ◆

10-Inch Homemade Blackberry-Blueberry Pie

(SERVES 8–10)

This was Jeff's favourite pie. He was tempted at times to have an extra slice despite the calories. This pie was a real morale booster for him on challenging days.

Leftover pie should be wrapped in plastic and kept chilled in the refrigerator.

DOUBLE CRUST PASTRY:

¾ cup + 2 tablespoons lard (or substitute 1 cup shortening)

2⅔ cups all-purpose flour

¾ teaspoon salt

8–9 tablespoons cold water

1. Combine flour and salt in a mixing bowl.
2. Cut in lard with a pastry cutter until mixture is crumbly.
3. Add water and mix well.
4. Knead dough by hand and gather into a large ball. Divide dough in half. Shape each half into a flattened round. Roll out pastry 1½ inches larger than inverted 10-inch pie plate with a floured rolling pin. Fold pastry in half and place in pie plate. Unfold pastry and pat against bottom and side of pie plate. Trim excess pastry with a knife.

FILLING:

2 cups fresh or frozen blackberries (antioxidant)

6 cups fresh or frozen blueberries (antioxidant)

1 cup white granulated sugar

½ cup + 1 tablespoon all-purpose flour

white granulated sugar, extra for sprinkling on top

1. Combine berries, sugar and flour in a large mixing bowl until fruit is well coated.
2. Spoon fruit mixture into pastry-lined 10-inch pie plate.

3. Place the other pastry crust on top. Trim excess pastry with a knife. Seal and flute edge with tines of fork. Cut four slits on top of crust with a knife.

4. Sprinkle extra sugar on top of crust.

5. Cover edge of pie with aluminum foil. Place pie on a large baking sheet.

6. Bake pie, on lower one-third of oven rack, in a preheated 425°F oven for 40 to 45 minutes. Remove foil during the last 15 minutes of baking. Broil 3 to 5 minutes more to brown the top of the pie.

◆ ◆ ◆

10-Inch Homemade Blueberry Pie
(SERVES 8–10)

This was one of our favourite pie recipes. Leftovers always vanished very quickly.

Leftover pie should be wrapped in plastic and kept chilled in the refrigerator.

DOUBLE CRUST PASTRY:

¾ cup + 2 tablespoons lard (or substitute 1 cup shortening)
2⅔ cups all-purpose flour
¾ teaspoon salt
8–9 tablespoons cold water

1. Combine flour and salt in a mixing bowl.
2. Cut in lard with a pastry cutter until mixture is crumbly.
3. Add water and mix well.
4. Knead dough by hand and gather into a large ball. Divide dough in half. Shape each half into a flattened round. Roll out pastry 1½ inches larger than inverted 10-inch pie plate with a floured rolling pin. Fold pastry in half and place in pie plate. Unfold pastry and pat against bottom and side of pie plate. Trim excess pastry with a knife.

FILLING:

8 cups fresh or frozen blueberries (antioxidant)
1 cup white granulated sugar
½ cup + 1 tablespoon all-purpose flour
white granulated sugar, extra for sprinkling on top

1. Combine berries, sugar and flour in a large mixing bowl until fruit is well coated.
2. Spoon fruit mixture into pastry-lined 10-inch pie plate.
3. Place the other pastry crust on top. Trim excess pastry with a knife. Seal and flute edge with tines of fork. Cut four slits on top of crust with a knife.

4. Sprinkle extra sugar on top of crust.

5. Cover edge of pie with aluminum foil. Place pie on a large baking sheet.

6. Bake pie, on lower one-third of oven rack, in a preheated 425°F oven for 40 to 45 minutes. Remove foil during the last 15 minutes of baking. Broil 3 to 5 minutes more to brown the top of the pie.

◆ ◆ ◆

Apple Crisp

(SERVES 8–10)

Jeff enjoyed this afternoon dessert most when it had been chilled in the refrigerator. This is a great way to get apples and oats in your diet.

6 cups Golden Delicious apples, scrubbed, cored and sliced
   (or substitute Granny Smith) (antioxidant)

sprinkle of nutmeg

juice of half a lemon (antioxidant)

1 cup quick cooking oats (antioxidant)

¾ cup all-purpose flour

¾ cup golden yellow sugar

⅓ cup margarine, softened at room temperature

1. Place apples in a 2-quart casserole or 8-inch square baking dish.
2. Sprinkle nutmeg and lemon juice on top.
3. Combine oats, flour and sugar in a mixing bowl.
4. Cut in margarine with a pastry cutter until mixture is crumbly. Sprinkle mixture evenly over fruit.
5. Bake, on middle oven rack, in a preheated 375°F oven for 30 to 35 minutes until golden brown.

◆ ◆ ◆

Fresh Fruit Salad

Jeff really enjoyed this healthy and low-fat fruit salad in the summer. This salad is very refreshing and full of antioxidants. It is a perfect accompaniment to any meal.

Leftover fruit salad can be stored in an airtight container in the refrigerator for a few days.

honeydew, seeded, peeled and cut into small chunks
cantaloupe, seeded, peeled and cut into small chunks (antioxidant)
seedless watermelon, peeled and cut into small chunks (antioxidant)
seedless red grapes, washed (antioxidant)
seedless green grapes, washed
strawberries, hulled, washed and halved (antioxidant)
raspberries, washed (antioxidant)
blueberries, washed (antioxidant)
juice of half a lemon (antioxidant)
1 tablespoon liquid honey

1. Combine prepared fruit in a large serving bowl until well mixed.
2. Sprinkle lemon juice and honey on top. Toss lightly to coat fruit.
3. Chill in refrigerator before serving.

◆ ◆ ◆

Fruity Dessert

(SERVES 4)

This quick dessert has a refreshing taste. The frozen berries and syrup give it an extra boost of flavour.

> 1 × 6 oz/85 g box of strawberry or raspberry jelly powder
> 1½ cups boiling water
> 10–12 oz container of frozen strawberries or raspberries with syrup, undrained (antioxidant)

1. Dissolve jelly powder in boiling water. Stir well.
2. Add frozen block of fruit and stir gently until fruit has separated.
3. Pour into a 5 cup/1.14L mould. Cover with lid and chill until firm for several hours or overnight.

◆ ◆ ◆

Mixed Fruit Dessert

(SERVES 8)

This refreshing dessert is a classic favourite with all ages.

1 × 170 g box of flavoured jelly powder (orange, lime, raspberry, strawberry or cherry flavour)

2 cups boiling water

2 cups cold water

2 medium sweet oranges, peeled and chopped (antioxidant)

1 large banana, peeled and diced

2 cups red or green seedless grapes, washed and dried (antioxidant)

1. Dissolve jelly powder in boiling water in a large mixing bowl.
2. Stir in cold water until well mixed.
3. Add prepared fruit and stir again.
4. Pour into a covered mould or serving bowl.
5. Chill in refrigerator at least 4 hours until set.

◆　◆　◆

Poached Allspice Pears

(SERVES 4)

This is a healthy and low-fat dessert. Allspice and raisins give the pears an extra boost of flavour.

Leftovers can be stored in an airtight container for 2 to 3 days.

> 4 large ripe pears, peeled, cored and halved
> 1¼ cups orange juice (antioxidant)
> 1 tablespoon ground allspice
> ⅓ cup sultana raisins
> 2 tablespoons golden yellow sugar

1. Place pear halves in a large saucepan.
2. Stir in remaining ingredients.
3. Cook over medium heat and stir until sugar is dissolved.
4. Bring mixture to a boil. Then reduce heat to low and simmer about 10 minutes or until the pears are cooked but still firm.
5. Remove pears with a slotted spoon and transfer to serving plates. Serve warm with extra syrup.

◆ ◆ ◆

EGGS, PANCAKES & WAFFLES

Eggs

Pancakes

Waffles

Boiled Eggs

(MAKES 4)

Jeff especially enjoyed his soft-boiled eggs with Homemade Belgian Waffles and maple syrup for breakfast. It was a wonderful way for him to start his mornings.

4 extra-large eggs, white or brown (antioxidant)

water

1. Place eggs in a medium saucepan. Cover eggs with cold water and lid.
2. Bring water to a boil over medium-high heat. Then lower to medium heat and cook 8 to 10 minutes for soft-boiled eggs, or 15 to 17 minutes for hard-boiled eggs.
3. Cool cooked eggs in a bowl of cold water before peeling.

◆ ◆ ◆

Pickled Eggs

(MAKES 12)

Jeff enjoyed these tangy pickled eggs as an afternoon treat while he was recovering from cancer treatments.

These eggs keep well for several months in a covered jar, if they last that long.

12 large hard-boiled eggs, shelled (antioxidant)

2 cups pure white vinegar

½ cup water

1 tablespoon salt

12 whole cloves

1 teaspoon whole black peppercorns

white vinegar, extra

1. Place prepared eggs in a large clean jar.
2. Pour 2 cups of vinegar and ½ cup of water in a medium saucepan. Add salt, cloves and peppercorns. Cook 10 minutes over medium heat. Let cool.
3. Remove cloves and peppercorns from saucepan with a slotted spoon. Pour cooled mixture over eggs.
4. Add extra vinegar to cover all of the eggs in the jar completely. Place lid on jar.
5. Let marinate in refrigerator at least 1 week before serving.

◆ ◆ ◆

Poached Eggs on English Muffins

(SERVES 2)

This is a healthy way to start off your morning. A glass of freshly squeezed orange juice goes well with this breakfast.

water

1½ tablespoons white vinegar

2 extra-large eggs (antioxidant)

dash of salt

freshly ground black pepper, to taste

1 whole extra crispy English muffin, halved and toasted

1. Fill a medium saucepan with enough water to cover the eggs fully.
2. Stir in vinegar.
3. Bring water and vinegar to a boil over medium-high heat. Then reduce heat to medium-low.
4. Gently break whole eggs in water. Cook eggs about 3 minutes or until set. Remove cooked eggs with a slotted spoon.
5. Serve eggs on English muffin halves. Season eggs with salt and black pepper.

◆ ◆ ◆

Scrambled Eggs

(MAKES 2)

Jeff enjoyed these scrambled eggs for breakfast. A glass of orange juice, rye toast with peanut butter and either honeydew or watermelon chunks completed this meal perfectly.

all-purpose cooking spray

4 extra-large eggs, beaten (antioxidant)

6 tablespoons skim milk (antioxidant)

dash of salt

freshly ground black pepper, to taste

1. Spray the bottom of a medium-size skillet with cooking spray.
2. Combine eggs, milk, salt and pepper in a bowl until well mixed.
3. Pour egg mixture into skillet.
4. Cook eggs over medium-high heat. Stir frequently until eggs are set.

◆ ◆ ◆

Turkey and Swiss Omelette

(SERVES 2–3)

This omelette was one of Jeff's favourite meals to start off the day. A glass of orange juice with calcium and fresh fruit chunks, such as watermelon or honeydew, were served with this meal.

all-purpose cooking spray

5 extra-large eggs, beaten well (antioxidant)

2½ tablespoons water

freshly ground black pepper, to taste

8 thin slices Swiss Emmenthal cheese

100 g thinly sliced deli turkey breast (or sun-dried tomato turkey breast, or deli chicken breast)

1. Spray the bottom of a 12-inch skillet with cooking spray.
2. Combine eggs, water and black pepper in a bowl until well mixed.
3. Pour egg mixture into skillet. Cook over medium heat. When edges of egg start to set, gently lift edges with a spatula so the uncooked portion of the egg flows underneath the cooked portion.
4. When eggs are almost set and cooked, place cheese slices in the middle of omelette.
5. Top with meat slices.
6. With a spatula, fold one-third of each side towards the middle of omelette so the edges overlap. Cook for 2 to 3 minutes. Flip omelette over carefully with a spatula and heat the other side for about 2 minutes more. Serve hot.

◆　◆　◆

Blueberry Cornmeal Pancakes

(SERVES 4)

These great-tasting pancakes are full of antioxidants. They are a healthy way to start your day.

Leftover pancakes can be stored in an airtight container in the refrigerator for up to 2 days. They can be reheated in the microwave.

1 cup all-purpose flour

2¼ tablespoons cornmeal

1 tablespoon white granulated sugar

1 teaspoon baking powder

½ teaspoon baking soda

dash of salt

dash of ground nutmeg

1 large egg, beaten (antioxidant)

1 cup skim milk (antioxidant) mixed with 1 tablespoon white vinegar, let stand for 5 minutes

2 tablespoons canola oil

1¼ cups frozen blueberries (antioxidant)

pure maple syrup

1. Combine the first seven ingredients in a large mixing bowl.
2. Add eggs, sour milk, oil and blueberries. Stir until just moistened and batter is still lumpy.
3. Pour ¼ of batter into 7½-inch skillet. Cook over medium heat for 3 to 4 minutes on each side until golden. Flip pancake over with a spatula when bubbly and edges are almost dry.
4. Serve pancakes with maple syrup.

◆ ◆ ◆

Spinach and Cheese Pancakes

(MAKES 3 LARGE)

This was Jeff's favourite pancake recipe for breakfast or lunch. He enjoyed these pancakes most while he was recovering from cancer treatments.

Leftover pancakes can be stored in an airtight container in the refrigerator for 2 to 3 days. They can be reheated in the microwave.

all-purpose cooking spray

1 × 300 g box frozen chopped spinach, cooked according to package directions, drained and squeezed dry (antioxidant)

½ cup all-purpose flour

pinch of salt

freshly ground black pepper, to taste

3 large eggs, beaten (antioxidant)

1 cup skim milk (antioxidant)

6 thin slices Swiss Emmenthal cheese (or white Cheddar cheese)

1. Spray the bottom of a 7½-inch skillet with cooking spray.
2. Mix together all ingredients, except cheese slices, in a large mixing bowl.
3. Pour ⅓ of batter into skillet and cook over medium heat. Top with 2 cheese slices.
4. When the bottom of pancake is set and golden (about 8 to 10 minutes), flip over with a spatula and cook until golden brown.

◆ ◆ ◆

Homemade Belgian Waffles

(MAKES 7 4-INCH SQUARES)

This was Jeff's favourite breakfast: large waffles that are crisp on the outside and tender on the inside. He enjoyed these waffles with maple syrup, soft-boiled eggs and orange juice on many mornings.

Leftover waffles can be stored in an airtight container in the refrigerator for 2 days. They can be reheated in the toaster.

1 cup all-purpose flour

1 teaspoon white granulated sugar

1 tablespoon baking powder

dash of salt

¼ cup canola oil

¾–1 cup skim milk (antioxidant)

1 large egg, beaten (antioxidant)

pure maple syrup

1. Heat Belgian waffle maker until ready to use.
2. Combine all ingredients, except maple syrup, in a mixing bowl. Beat until batter is smooth and lump free.
3. Pour batter into hot waffle maker. Close the lid.
4. Cook 7 to 8 minutes until waffles are golden brown.
5. Serve hot with maple syrup.

◆ ◆ ◆

SOUPS & STEWS

Soups

Stews

Chicken and Corn Soup

(SERVES 6–8)

This sweet and creamy soup has been a family favourite over the years.

Leftover soup can be stored in a covered container in the refrigerator. It is just as tasty the next day when you reheat it in the microwave.

1 whole skinless and boneless chicken breast, chopped finely

1 teaspoon cornstarch

2 × 10 oz/284 mL cans chicken broth

1¾ soup cans of water

3 tablespoons cornstarch, mixed with 1 tablespoon water

3 × 14 oz/398 mL cans cream corn

1 tablespoon dry sherry

1 tablespoon dark soy sauce

3 large beaten eggs (antioxidant)

1. Combine chicken with 1 teaspoon cornstarch in a bowl. Set aside.
2. Bring chicken broth and water in a large pot to a boil over high heat.
3. Stir in remaining cornstarch mixture.
4. Add chicken mixture, corn, sherry and soy sauce. Reduce heat to medium, cover with lid and cook 15 minutes, stirring occasionally.
5. Stir in beaten eggs and cook another 5 minutes.

◆ ◆ ◆

Crab Soup

(SERVES 6)

This is another recipe that has been a family favourite over the years. The shiitake mushrooms give this soup an Asian flavour.

Any leftover soup is best stored in a covered container in the refrigerator. It can be reheated in the microwave the following day.

3½ cups chicken broth

2½ cups water

4 chopped green onions (antioxidant)

4 dried shiitake mushrooms, soaked in boiling water 40 minutes, squeezed
    dry, stems removed and sliced thinly (antioxidant)

2 × 4 oz/120 g cans crabmeat, drained and flaked with a fork

4 tablespoons cornstarch mixed with 1 tablespoon water

1½ tablespoons dark soy sauce

dash of dry sherry

salt, to taste

freshly ground black pepper, to taste

3 large beaten egg whites mixed with 2 tablespoons water

1. Bring chicken broth and water in a large pot to a boil over medium-high heat.
2. Stir in remaining ingredients except egg mixture. Bring to a boil again.
   Then reduce heat to medium and cook 5 to 6 minutes.
3. Stir in egg mixture slowly. Cook another 2 to 3 minutes.

◆ ◆ ◆

Karen's Hot and Sour Soup

(SERVES 6)

This spicy soup is loaded with antioxidants from mushrooms and tofu. Jeff enjoyed this soup best while he was recovering from cancer treatments.

Leftover soup is best stored in a covered container in the refrigerator for 2 to 3 days. It can be reheated in the microwave.

12 dried shiitake mushrooms, soaked in boiling water 40 minutes, squeezed dry, stems removed and sliced thinly (antioxidant)

1 grated carrot (antioxidant)

4 large dried fungi, soaked in hot water 30 minutes, rinsed and sliced thinly

1 × 700 g package traditional or smooth tofu cubes, drained and sliced lengthwise (antioxidant)

⅓ cup sliced bamboo shoots

¼–½ teaspoon dried chili flakes

2 × 14½ oz cans chicken broth

3 cups water

10 tablespoons red wine vinegar

6 tablespoons pure white vinegar

1 tablespoon dark soy sauce

dash of salt

dash of white pepper

1 teaspoon ground chili paste

4 tablespoons cornstarch mixed with 2½ teaspoons water

1 large beaten egg (antioxidant)

1. Combine all ingredients, except cornstarch mixture and beaten egg, in a large pot.
2. Bring to a boil over medium-high heat. Then reduce heat to medium and cook 20 to 25 minutes.
3. Stir in cornstarch mixture and beaten egg.
4. Cook another 10 minutes.

◆ ◆ ◆

Split Pea Soup

(SERVES 12)

This has been our favourite pea soup recipe over the years. It is great comfort food for the winter months. A chunk of freshly-baked bread is a perfect accompaniment to this soup at lunch or dinner.

Leftover soup is best stored in a covered container in the refrigerator for up to 3 days. It also freezes well in freezer containers for several months.

2½ cups dried split green peas (antioxidant)

8½ cups cold water

salt, to taste

freshly ground black pepper, to taste

2–2½ cups smoked boneless ham, chopped finely

1. Bring all ingredients in a large pot to a boil over medium heat.
2. Reduce heat to medium-low, cover and cook about 2 hours until peas are tender.

◆ ◆ ◆

Tomato Clam Chowder

(SERVES 6–7)

This easy-to-make soup is nutritious and filling. It is full of antioxidants and it makes a fabulous meal when served with a whole wheat bun at lunch.

Leftover soup is best stored in a covered container in the refrigerator for up to 3 days. This soup freezes well for up to 3 months in freezer containers.

> 2 × 142 g cans whole baby clams with juices
>
> 3–4 cups peeled and chopped potatoes (antioxidant)
>
> 1 celery stalk, diced (antioxidant)
>
> dash of dried thyme leaves (optional)
>
> salt, to taste
>
> freshly ground black pepper, to taste
>
> 1 × 28 oz/796 mL can whole tomatoes with juices, cut up (antioxidant)

1. Bring all ingredients in a large pot to a boil over medium-high heat.
2. Reduce heat to medium-low, cover with lid and cook 15 to 20 minutes until potatoes are tender.

◆ ◆ ◆

Dark and Delicious Homemade Chili

(SERVES 6–8)

This was Jeff's favourite chili, which he often enjoyed with a chunk of freshly-baked whole wheat bread while recovering from cancer treatments. It is loaded with antioxidants.

Leftover chili is best stored in an airtight container in the refrigerator for up to 3 days. This recipe freezes well in freezer containers for several months.

2 lbs lean ground beef

1 medium onion, peeled and chopped (antioxidant)

1½ cups celery, chopped finely (antioxidant)

2 medium green bell peppers, chopped (antioxidant) (optional)

2½ tablespoons premium cocoa powder

1½ tablespoons all-purpose flour

1 teaspoon white granulated sugar

dash of garlic powder

1½ tablespoons chili powder

1½ teaspoons dried oregano leaves

1 teaspoon salt

1¼ tablespoons curry powder (antioxidant)

½ teaspoon dried crushed chilies

2 × 28 oz/796 mL cans whole tomatoes, cut up with juices (antioxidant)

2 × 19 oz/540 mL cans red kidney beans, undrained (antioxidant)

1. Crumble beef in a large pot.
2. Cook beef with onion over medium heat until meat is no longer pink inside. Drain fat.
3. Stir in remaining ingredients, except beans, and bring mixture to a boil. Then reduce heat to medium-low, cover and cook for 40 minutes, stirring twice.
4. Stir in kidney beans and cook for another 15 minutes.

◆ ◆ ◆

Easy Beef Stew

(SERVES 10–12)

This quick stew is comfort food in the fall and winter months. A green salad and a whole wheat bun make this stew part of a nutritious dinner.

Leftover stew is best stored in an airtight container in the refrigerator for up to 3 days. This recipe freezes well in freezer containers for several months.

> all-purpose cooking spray
>
> 3 lbs top sirloin roast, cut into 1-inch cubes
>
> ½ cup all-purpose flour
>
> salt, to taste
>
> freshly ground black pepper, to taste
>
> 1 × 28 oz/796 mL can sliced stewed tomatoes (antioxidant)
>
> 1 × 10 oz/284 mL can condensed beef consommé
>
> ½ cup water
>
> 6 medium carrots, cut into 1-inch chunks (antioxidant)
>
> 4 medium potatoes, peeled and cut into 1-inch chunks (antioxidant)
>
> 1 teaspoon dried thyme

1. Spray the bottom of a large pot with all-purpose cooking spray.
2. Toss and coat meat in flour.
3. Brown meat mixture over medium heat.
4. Season with salt and pepper.
5. Stir in remaining ingredients and bring to a boil. Reduce heat to medium-low, cover and simmer for 1 hour.

◆ ◆ ◆

Hungarian Goulash

(SERVES 8–10)

This was Jeff's favourite goulash, especially when served with a chunk of freshly-baked whole wheat bread. It is loaded with antioxidants, but this spicy recipe is more suitable between cancer treatments.

Leftover goulash is best stored in an airtight container in the refrigerator for up to 3 days. This recipe freezes well in freezer containers for several months.

    1 tablespoon extra virgin olive oil (antioxidant)

    1 large onion, chopped (antioxidant)

    2 cloves garlic, peeled and minced (antioxidant) (or substitute ½ teaspoon
        garlic powder)

    4½ tablespoons Hungarian paprika

    2½ lbs lean beef sirloin, cut into 1-inch cubes

    4 cups chicken broth

    salt, to taste

    freshly ground black pepper, to taste

    4–5 large russet potatoes, peeled and cut into 1½-inch cubes (antioxidant)

    4 large tomatoes, cut into chunks (antioxidant)

    2 medium green bell peppers, seeded and cut into chunks (antioxidant)

    1 teaspoon dried marjoram leaves

1. Heat oil in a large pot over medium heat.
2. Add onion and garlic. Sauté until softened. Remove from heat.
3. Stir in paprika.
4. Return to heat and add beef, broth, salt and pepper. Bring to a boil. Reduce heat to medium-low and simmer, covered, about 1 hour.
5. Add potatoes, tomatoes, green peppers and marjoram. Cook another 1¾ hours.

◆ ◆ ◆

SANDWICHES

Chicken Salad on Toasted Rye

(SERVES 3)

This is one of our favourite sandwiches. The celery gives an added crunch in this sandwich.

1 ¼ cups cooked chicken breast meat, chopped

⅓ cup celery, chopped (antioxidant)

¼ cup light salad dressing (or mayonnaise)

salt, to taste

freshly ground black pepper, to taste

6 slices toasted rye bread

1. Mix together the first five ingredients in a bowl.
2. Spread chicken salad filling between two slices of bread.
3. Cut each sandwich in half with a sharp knife.

◆ ◆ ◆

Egg Salad Sandwiches

(SERVES 4)

This recipe is a healthy alternative to meat sandwiches.

Leftover sandwiches can be stored in an airtight container in the refrigerator, but they should be eaten the next day.

6–7 large hard-boiled eggs, shelled and chopped (antioxidant)

⅓ cup light salad dressing (or mayonnaise)

2 green onions, chopped (antioxidant)

salt, to taste

freshly ground black pepper, to taste

alfalfa sprouts, rinsed and drained well

8 slices toasted rye bread

1. Mix together eggs, dressing, onions, salt and pepper in a bowl.
2. Place alfalfa sprouts on 4 slices of bread.
3. Spread ¼ of egg mixture on top.
4. Top with remaining 4 slices of bread.
5. Cut each sandwich in half with a sharp knife.

◆ ◆ ◆

Grilled Cheese Sandwiches

(SERVES 2)

This is an ideal recipe to make when you do not require meat at lunch.

all-purpose cooking spray
4 slices 100% whole wheat or multigrain bread
2 slices light medium Cheddar cheese
2 dill pickles, sliced lengthwise in thirds

1. Spray the bottom of a skillet or frying pan with all-purpose cooking spray.
2. Place cheese slice between 2 slices of bread.
3. Grill sandwiches in skillet over medium heat until golden brown on both sides and cheese is melted, about 6 to 7 minutes total.
4. Serve hot with sliced pickles.

◆　◆　◆

Grilled Ham and Cheese Sandwiches

(SERVES 2)

The combination of Black Forest ham and Swiss cheese gives these sandwiches a rich and smoky flavour.

all-purpose cooking spray

4 slices rye bread

4 thin slices cooked Black Forest ham

2 thin slices Swiss cheese (or mozzarella cheese (antioxidant)**)**

1. Spray the bottom of a large skillet or frying pan with all-purpose cooking spray.
2. Place two slices of ham and one slice of cheese between 2 slices of bread.
3. Grill sandwiches on both sides in skillet over medium heat until golden brown and cheese is melted, about 6 to 7 minutes total.
4. Cut each sandwich in half with a sharp knife.

◆　◆　◆

Grilled Turkey and Swiss Sandwiches

(SERVES 2)

This has been one of our favourite sandwiches over the years. Turkey breast and Swiss cheese slices go well together in this recipe.

all-purpose cooking spray

4 slices multigrain bread (or 100% whole wheat)

4–6 thin slices deli turkey breast

2 thin slices Swiss cheese

1. Spray the bottom of a large skillet or frying pan with all-purpose cooking spray.
2. Place meat and cheese between 2 slices of bread.
3. Grill sandwiches on both sides over medium heat until golden brown and cheese is melted, about 6 to 7 minutes total.
4. Cut sandwiches in half with a sharp knife.

◆ ◆ ◆

Hummus Alfalfa Pita Pockets

(MAKES 6)

This is a very healthy, low-fat vegetarian sandwich. This recipe can be halved, if desired.

2 cups prepared hummus dip

6 whole wheat pita pockets

6 medium tomatoes, seeded and chopped (antioxidant)

alfalfa sprouts, washed and drained well

1. Spread hummus on one side of each pita pocket.
2. Top with tomatoes and alfalfa sprouts.

◆ ◆ ◆

Salmon Salad on Toasted Rye

(SERVES 2)

This was Jeff's favourite sandwich during cancer treatments and post-treatment recovery. He left no crumbs on his plate when he enjoyed this sandwich with a glass of apple juice and a serving of watermelon chunks.

1 × 7½ oz/213 g can sockeye salmon, drained (antioxidant)

1 stalk celery, chopped (antioxidant)

salt, to taste

freshly ground black pepper, to taste

light salad dressing (or mayonnaise)

dash of lemon juice (optional) (antioxidant)

4 slices rye bread, toasted

dill pickles, sliced

pickled asparagus spears (antioxidant)

1. Mix together the first six ingredients in a bowl until well blended.
2. Spread salmon mixture on 2 slices of bread. Top with remaining 2 slices of bread.
3. Cut sandwiches in half with a sharp knife.
4. Serve with pickles and asparagus spears.

◆ ◆ ◆

Shrimp and Avocado Croissants
(SERVES 4)

This is a great summer recipe, if you don't mind the extra calories.

light salad dressing (or mayonnaise)

4 croissants, halved lengthwise

4 green leaf lettuce leaves (or iceberg lettuce)

2 medium tomatoes, sliced in 12s (antioxidant)

½ lb cooked shrimp, drained well

1 large ripe avocado, pitted, peeled and sliced in 12s (antioxidant)

salt, to taste

freshly ground black pepper, to taste

1. Spread dressing on bottom of each croissant.
2. Place lettuce, tomatoes, shrimp and avocado slices on top.
3. Top with remaining croissant halves.
4. Cut croissants in half with a sharp knife.

◆ ◆ ◆

BREADS, CALZONES & PIZZAS

Breads

Calzones

Pizzas

Banana Bread

(MAKES 2 LOAVES/32 SLICES)

This banana bread recipe is a long-time family favourite. It is a great way to use overripe bananas.

This bread freezes well, so you can make one to eat now and freeze the other to enjoy later, if desired.

3 cups all-purpose flour

1½ cups white granulated sugar

2¾ teaspoons baking powder

1 teaspoon baking soda

sprinkle of ground nutmeg

dash of salt

2 large eggs, beaten (antioxidant)

6 medium (about 2 cups) very ripe bananas, mashed

½ cup canola oil

1. Combine all ingredients in a large mixing bowl. Stir until well blended.
2. Pour batter into two 8×4×2-inch loaf pans. Spread evenly with a wooden spoon.
3. Bake, on middle oven rack, in a preheated 350°F oven for 50 to 60 minutes until a wooden toothpick inserted near the centre comes out clean.

♦ ♦ ♦

Easy Cheese Bread

(MAKES 1 LOAF/10–12 SLICES)

This is the best cheese bread you will ever taste.

It should be stored in an airtight container in the refrigerator for a few days. Leftover bread can be reheated in the toaster.

2 cups all-purpose flour

1 tablespoon white granulated sugar

2¼ tablespoons baking powder

1 teaspoon dry mustard

¼ teaspoon salt

¼ cup margarine, melted

1 large egg, beaten (antioxidant)

¾ cup skim milk (antioxidant)

2½ cups aged Cheddar cheese, grated (or Asiago cheese)

1. Combine all ingredients in a large mixing bowl. Stir until well mixed.
2. Pour batter into an 8½×4½×2-inch loaf pan. Spread evenly with a wooden spoon.
3. Bake, on middle oven rack, in a preheated 350°F oven for 45 minutes.

◆ ◆ ◆

Pepperoni Calzones

(MAKES 6)

You will not find a calzone recipe like this one. It is always a success.

Any leftovers can be stored in a covered container in the refrigerator for 2 to 3 days. The calzones can be reheated in the microwave the following day.

1 tablespoon white granulated sugar

1 cup hot water

1¼ tablespoons active dry yeast

2 tablespoons extra virgin olive oil (antioxidant)

½ teaspoon salt

3–3¼ cups all-purpose flour

1 cup/8 oz all-purpose tomato sauce (antioxidant)

½ cup canned sliced mushrooms, drained

1 teaspoon dried basil leaves

1 teaspoon dried oregano leaves

dash of garlic powder

1½–1⅔ cups thinly sliced pepperoni sticks (about 3 sticks)

1¼–1⅓ cups mozzarella cheese, shredded (antioxidant)

1 large egg, beaten (antioxidant)

1. Dissolve sugar in hot water in a bowl. Stir well.
2. Sprinkle yeast on top. Let stand 10 minutes until foamy.
3. Combine oil, salt and flour in a large mixing bowl until well mixed. Knead dough by hand until smooth and elastic and gather into a large ball. Place dough in a bowl and cover with plastic wrap and a tea towel. Let rise ½ hour in a warm place until doubled in size.
4. Punch down risen dough. Divide into six equal portions. Roll each portion into a 7-inch circle with a floured rolling pin.
5. Mix together tomato sauce, mushrooms, basil, oregano and garlic powder in a separate bowl. Spread over half of each circle to within one inch of edge.

6. Top with pepperoni and cheese. Fold dough over filling. Pinch edges to seal. Let stand on baking sheet for 30 to 45 minutes until risen again.

7. Brush tops of calzones with egg.

8. Bake calzones, on middle oven rack, in a preheated 375°F oven for 30 to 35 minutes until golden brown.

◆ ◆ ◆

Karen's 15-Inch Beef and Sausage Pizza
(SERVES 8–10)

This spicy pizza is not low in fat or calories, but Jeff enjoyed this pizza at lunch while he was recovering from cancer treatments.

Leftover pizza is best stored in a covered container in the refrigerator for 2 to 3 days. It freezes well in freezer containers for up to 2 months.

PIZZA CRUST:

¼ cup warm water

1 teaspoon white granulated sugar

1½ tablespoons active dry yeast

2½ cups all-purpose flour

1 teaspoon salt

2 tablespoons extra virgin olive oil (antioxidant)

¾ cup hot boiled water, cooled 2 minutes

4½ tablespoons cornmeal

all-purpose cooking spray

1. Dissolve sugar in ¼ cup warm water in a bowl. Stir well.
2. Sprinkle yeast on top. Let stand 10 minutes until foamy.
3. Combine flour, salt, oil and ¾ cup hot water in a large mixing bowl until well mixed.
4. Stir in prepared yeast mixture. Knead dough by hand until smooth and elastic. Gather into a large ball. Place dough in a large bowl and cover with plastic wrap and a tea towel. Let rise in a warm place until light and doubled in size about 45 minutes.
5. Spray a 16-inch pizza pan with all-purpose cooking spray.
6. Punch down risen dough several times to remove air bubbles.
7. Add cornmeal and knead dough again. Gather into a large ball and shape into a flattened round. Place on pizza pan. Roll dough out to 15 inches with a floured rolling pin. Prick crust all over with the tines of a fork.

8. Bake pizza crust, on bottom oven rack, in a preheated 425°F oven for 15 minutes.

9. Top with the following ingredients in the order listed below. Bake an additional 15 minutes until crust is golden brown and toppings are heated. Broil 3 minutes more to brown cheese on top.

TOPPINGS:

¼ cup all-purpose tomato sauce (antioxidant)

1 teaspoon dried basil leaves

1½ teaspoons dried oregano leaves

1 lb lean ground beef, cooked, drained and crumbled

1 large wine chorizo sausage, cooked, drained and crumbled

⅛ cup bacon bits

⅓ cup cooked sliced mushrooms, drained well

⅓ cup ripe black olives, sliced

1 small green or red bell pepper, seeded and sliced thinly (antioxidant)

1 small white onion, peeled and diced (antioxidant)

1⅔ cups Feta cheese, crumbled (or grated Marble cheese)

10–12 thin slices of pepper salami

◆ ◆ ◆

Karen's 15-Inch Deluxe Pizza

(SERVES 8–10)

This was Jeff's favourite pizza recipe. While it is not low in fat or calories, he still enjoyed this pizza at lunch while he was recuperating from cancer treatments.

Leftover pizza is best stored in a covered container in the refrigerator for 2 to 3 days. It freezes well in freezer containers for up to 2 months.

PIZZA CRUST:

¼ cup warm water

1 teaspoon white granulated sugar

1½ tablespoons active dry yeast

2½ cups all-purpose flour

1 teaspoon salt

2 tablespoons extra virgin olive oil (antioxidant)

¾ cup hot boiled water, cooled 2 minutes

4½ tablespoons cornmeal

all-purpose cooking spray

1. Dissolve sugar in ¼ cup warm water in a bowl. Stir well.
2. Sprinkle yeast on top. Let stand 10 minutes until foamy.
3. Combine flour, salt, oil and ¾ cup hot water in a large mixing bowl until well mixed.
4. Stir in prepared yeast mixture. Knead dough by hand until smooth and elastic. Gather into a large ball. Place dough in a large bowl and cover with plastic wrap and a tea towel. Let rise in a warm place until light and doubled in size about 45 minutes.
5. Spray a 16-inch pizza pan with all-purpose cooking spray.
6. Punch down risen dough several times to remove air bubbles.
7. Add cornmeal and knead dough again. Gather into a large ball and shape into a flattened round. Place on pizza pan. Roll dough out to 15 inches with a floured rolling pin. Prick crust all over with the tines of a fork.

8. Bake pizza crust, on bottom oven rack, in a preheated 425°F oven for 15 minutes.

9. Top with the following ingredients in the order listed below. Bake an additional 15 minutes until crust is golden brown and toppings are heated. Broil 3 minutes more to brown cheese on top.

TOPPINGS:

¼ cup all-purpose tomato sauce (antioxidant)

1 teaspoon dried basil leaves

1½ teaspoons dried oregano leaves

2 hot Italian sausages, cooked, drained and crumbled

2 pepperoni sticks, cut into small chunks

⅛ cup bacon bits

⅓ cup ripe black olives, sliced

1 small green or red bell pepper, seeded and sliced thinly (antioxidant)

1 small red onion, peeled and sliced thinly (antioxidant)

¾ cup unsweetened pineapple chunks, drained well (antioxidant)

1⅔ cups light mozzarella cheese, grated (antioxidant)

10–12 thin slices of pepper salami

◆ ◆ ◆

Karen's 15-Inch Ham and Pineapple Pizza

(SERVES 8–10)

This recipe is a family favourite and is lower in fat and calories than the other pizzas in this book.

Leftover pizza is best stored in a covered container in the refrigerator for 2 to 3 days. This recipe freezes well in freezer containers for up to 2 months.

PIZZA CRUST:

¼ cup warm water

1 teaspoon white granulated sugar

1½ tablespoons active dry yeast

2½ cups all-purpose flour

1 teaspoon salt

2 tablespoons extra virgin olive oil (antioxidant)

¾ cup hot boiled water, cooled 2 minutes

4½ tablespoons cornmeal

all-purpose cooking spray

1. Dissolve sugar in ¼ cup warm water in a bowl. Stir well.

2. Sprinkle yeast on top. Let stand 10 minutes until foamy.

3. Combine flour, salt, oil and ¾ cup hot water in a large mixing bowl until well mixed.

4. Stir in prepared yeast mixture. Knead dough by hand until smooth and elastic. Gather into a large ball. Place dough in a large bowl and cover with plastic wrap and a tea towel. Let rise in a warm place until light and doubled in size about 45 minutes.

5. Spray a 16-inch pizza pan with all-purpose cooking spray.

6. Punch down risen dough several times to remove air bubbles.

7. Add cornmeal and knead dough again. Gather into a large ball and shape into a flattened round. Place on pizza pan. Roll dough out to 15 inches with a floured rolling pin. Prick crust all over with the tines of a fork.

8. Bake pizza crust, on bottom oven rack, in a preheated 425°F oven for 15 minutes.
9. Top with the following ingredients in the order listed below. Bake an additional 15 minutes until crust is golden brown and toppings are heated. Broil 3 minutes more to brown cheese on top.

TOPPINGS:

¼ cup all-purpose tomato sauce (antioxidant)

1 teaspoon dried basil leaves

1½ teaspoons dried oregano leaves

2–2½ lbs cooked smoked ham, diced

⅓ cup ripe black olives, sliced

⅓ cup cooked sliced mushrooms, drained well

1 small green bell pepper, seeded and sliced thinly (antioxidant)

1 small red onion, peeled and sliced thinly (antioxidant)

¾ cup unsweetened pineapple chunks, drained well (antioxidant)

1⅔ cups light medium Cheddar cheese, grated
    (or light mozzarella cheese (antioxidant))

10–12 thin slices of pepper salami

◆ ◆ ◆

Karen's 15-Inch Ham and Shrimp Pizza
(SERVES 8–10)

This pizza is a nice change from other recipes. Black Forest ham and shrimp make a fantastic combination in this recipe.

Leftover pizza is best stored in a covered container in the refrigerator for 2 to 3 days. It freezes well in freezer containers for up to 2 months.

PIZZA CRUST:

¼ cup warm water

1 teaspoon white granulated sugar

1½ tablespoons active dry yeast

2½ cups all-purpose flour

1 teaspoon salt

2 tablespoons extra virgin olive oil (antioxidant)

¾ cup hot boiled water, cooled 2 minutes

4½ tablespoons cornmeal

all-purpose cooking spray

1. Dissolve sugar in ¼ cup warm water in a bowl. Stir well.
2. Sprinkle yeast on top. Let stand 10 minutes until foamy.
3. Combine flour, salt, oil and ¾ cup hot water in a large mixing bowl until well mixed.
4. Stir in prepared yeast mixture. Knead dough by hand until smooth and elastic. Gather into a large ball. Place dough in a large bowl and cover with plastic wrap and a tea towel. Let rise in a warm place until light and doubled in size about 45 minutes.
5. Spray a 16-inch pizza pan with all-purpose cooking spray.
6. Punch down risen dough several times to remove air bubbles.
7. Add cornmeal and knead dough again. Gather into a large ball and shape into a flattened round. Place on pizza pan. Roll dough out to 15 inches with a floured rolling pin. Prick crust all over with the tines of a fork.

8. Bake pizza crust, on bottom oven rack, in a preheated 425°F oven for 15 minutes.

9. Top with the following ingredients in the order listed below. Bake an additional 15 minutes until crust is golden brown and toppings are heated. Broil 3 minutes more to brown cheese on top.

TOPPINGS:

¼ cup all-purpose tomato sauce (antioxidant)

1 teaspoon dried basil leaves

1½ teaspoons dried oregano leaves

2 lbs Black Forest ham, cooked and diced

½ lb cooked shrimp

⅓ cup ripe black olives, sliced

1 small green bell pepper, seeded and sliced thinly (antioxidant)

1 small red onion, peeled and sliced thinly (antioxidant)

¾ cup unsweetened pineapple chunks, drained well (antioxidant)

1⅔ cups Marble cheese, grated (light cheese preferred)

10–12 thin slices of pepper salami

◆ ◆ ◆

Karen's 15-Inch Turkey and Cheese Pizza

(SERVES 8–10)

This pizza is lower in fat and calories compared to other recipes in this book.

Leftover pizza can be stored in a covered container in the refrigerator for 2 to 3 days, if it lasts that long.

PIZZA CRUST:

¼ cup warm water

1 teaspoon white granulated sugar

1½ tablespoons active dry yeast

2½ cups all-purpose flour

1 teaspoon salt

2 tablespoons extra virgin olive oil (antioxidant)

¾ cup hot boiled water, cooled 2 minutes

4½ tablespoons cornmeal

all-purpose cooking spray

1. Dissolve sugar in ¼ cup warm water in a bowl. Stir well.
2. Sprinkle yeast on top. Let stand 10 minutes until foamy.
3. Combine flour, salt, oil and ¾ cup hot water in a large mixing bowl until well mixed.
4. Stir in prepared yeast mixture. Knead dough by hand until smooth and elastic. Gather into a large ball. Place dough in a large bowl and cover with plastic wrap and a tea towel. Let rise in a warm place until light and doubled in size about 45 minutes.
5. Spray a 16-inch pizza pan with all-purpose cooking spray.
6. Punch down risen dough several times to remove air bubbles.
7. Add cornmeal and knead dough again. Gather into a large ball and shape into a flattened round. Place on pizza pan. Roll dough out to 15 inches with a floured rolling pin. Prick crust all over with the tines of a fork.

8. Bake pizza crust, on bottom oven rack, in a preheated 425°F oven for 15 minutes.

9. Top with the following ingredients in the order listed below. Bake an additional 15 minutes until crust is golden brown and toppings are heated. Broil 3 minutes more to brown cheese on top.

TOPPINGS:

¼ **cup all-purpose tomato sauce** (antioxidant)

1 **teaspoon dried basil leaves**

1½ **teaspoons dried oregano leaves**

300 g **cooked deli turkey breast slices**

⅓ **cup ripe black olives, sliced**

1 **small green or red bell pepper, seeded and sliced thinly** (antioxidant)

1 **small red onion, peeled and sliced thinly** (antioxidant)

¾ **cup unsweetened pineapple chunks, drained well** (antioxidant)

1⅔ **cups smoked white Cheddar cheese, grated (or aged Cheddar)**

◆ ◆ ◆

SALADS

Great Caesar Salad

(SERVES 6)

This was one of Jeff's favourite salads, which he enjoyed while recuperating from cancer treatments.

Leftover salad can be stored in an airtight container in the refrigerator. It should be eaten the next day.

DRESSING:

6 cloves garlic, peeled and sliced lengthwise into quarters (antioxidant)
1 cup extra virgin olive oil (antioxidant)

1. Combine garlic and oil in a covered jar.
2. Refrigerate at least 24 hours before removing garlic pieces and using dressing.

SALAD:

1 large head romaine lettuce, washed and torn into bite-size pieces
2 tablespoons red wine vinegar
juice of half a lemon (antioxidant)
2 large eggs (antioxidant)
dash of Worcestershire sauce
dash of salt
generous sprinkle of freshly ground black pepper
⅓ cup grated Parmesan cheese
1 cup lightly seasoned croutons
1 × 50 g tin flat anchovy fillets in olive oil, drained and chopped

1. Place torn lettuce in a large serving bowl.
2. Drizzle with ⅓ cup of prepared dressing.
3. Sprinkle red wine vinegar on top.

4. Squeeze juice of lemon all over lettuce.

5. Place whole eggs in a saucepan of boiling water and let stand 1 minute. Cool eggs slightly and then break them over lettuce leaves.

6. Add Worcestershire, salt, pepper, Parmesan, croutons and anchovies.

7. Toss salad lightly with a serving fork and a spoon until well coated with dressing.

◆ ◆ ◆

Mexican Corn and Bean Salad

(SERVES 6)

This summer salad is loaded with antioxidants and a perfect accompaniment to grilled meat on the barbecue.

Leftover salad can be stored in a covered container in the refrigerator for a few days.

2 cups red kidney beans, drained well (antioxidant)

1 cup whole kernel corn, drained well

½ cup green bell pepper, diced (antioxidant)

½ cup red bell pepper, diced (antioxidant)

2 tablespoons extra virgin olive oil (antioxidant)

3 tablespoons red wine vinegar

salt, to taste

freshly ground black pepper, to taste

1. Mix together all ingredients in a serving bowl until well blended.
2. Chill before serving.

❖ ❖ ❖

Potato and Egg Salad

(SERVES 10)

This is one of our favourite salads for summer picnics. This recipe can be halved, if desired.

Leftover salad can be stored in a covered container in the refrigerator. It should be eaten within 2 to 3 days.

6–7 medium potatoes, cooked, peeled and cubed (antioxidant)

1–1½ cups fat-free salad dressing (or mayonnaise)

3–4 dill pickles, chopped

2 tablespoons pickle juice

salt, to taste

freshly ground black pepper, to taste

4–5 large hard-boiled eggs, shelled and chopped (antioxidant)

2 stalks green onions, chopped (antioxidant)

1. Combine all ingredients in a large serving bowl. Mix well.
2. Cover and refrigerate for 4 hours before serving.

◆ ◆ ◆

Quick Caesar Salad

(SERVES 6)

This is another one of our favourite salads. Jeff really enjoyed it while he was recovering from cancer treatments. This recipe comes in handy when you have limited time to cook.

Leftover salad can be stored in an airtight container in the refrigerator. It is best eaten the next day.

> 1 head romaine lettuce, washed and torn into bite-size pieces
> ½–¾ cup lightly seasoned croutons
> 1 × 50 g can anchovy fillets in olive oil, drained and chopped
> freshly ground coarse black pepper, to taste
> juice of 1 lemon (antioxidant)
> ½ cup light Caesar dressing

1. Mix together all ingredients in a large serving bowl.
2. Refrigerate salad for 1 hour before serving.

◆ ◆ ◆

Quick Greek Salad

(SERVES 6)

This was Jeff's favourite Mediterranean salad for many years. It is loaded with antioxidants. He particularly enjoyed this salad at lunch with a sandwich or at dinner with a chicken dish.

Leftover salad can be stored in a covered container in the refrigerator for 3 to 4 days.

5–6 medium Roma tomatoes, cut into bite-size wedges (antioxidant)

1 small cucumber, peeled and cut into bite-size chunks

1 medium green bell pepper, cut into bite-size chunks (antioxidant)

1 medium red onion, cut into small chunks (antioxidant)

½ cup Kalamata olives

¾–1 cup Greek Feta cheese, crumbled

2 tablespoons extra virgin olive oil (antioxidant)

2 tablespoons balsamic vinegar (high-quality brand preferred)

1. Combine the first five ingredients in a large salad bowl.
2. Sprinkle crumbled cheese on top.
3. Drizzle with oil and vinegar.
4. Chill at least 2 to 3 hours for flavours to blend. Toss well just before serving.

◆ ◆ ◆

Spinach and Mandarin Salad

(SERVES 4–5)

This is a refreshing salad to serve in the summer months. The sweetness from the jam and the tanginess from the red wine vinegar go well together. Also, this salad is loaded with antioxidants.

Leftover salad can be stored in a covered container in the refrigerator. It is best eaten the next day.

1 bunch baby spinach leaves, washed and dried in a salad spinner (antioxidant)

1 small can mandarin orange segments, juice drained (antioxidant)

1 small red onion, peeled and sliced thinly (antioxidant)

2 tablespoons orange marmalade jam

4 tablespoons red wine vinegar

1 tablespoon extra virgin olive oil (antioxidant)

1. Combine spinach, orange and onion in a large salad bowl.
2. Mix together jam, vinegar and oil in a small bowl.
3. Pour dressing over salad. Toss well to coat.
4. Chill at least 1 hour before serving.

◆ ◆ ◆

Super Spinach, Egg and Bacon Salad
(SERVES 8)

This was one of Jeff's favourite salad recipes. He always had a generous second helping. Some advance preparation is required; however, this salad is worth the effort.

Leftover salad is best stored in a covered container in the refrigerator. It should be eaten the next day.

DRESSING:

½ cup extra virgin olive oil (antioxidant)

⅛ cup pure white vinegar

juice of 1 lemon (antioxidant)

dash of salt

¼ teaspoon dry mustard

¼ teaspoon paprika

1 clove garlic, peeled and halved lengthwise (antioxidant)

1. Combine the first six ingredients in a small bowl. Stir well.
2. Let garlic halves stand in dressing for 1½ to 2 hours before using.

SALAD:

1½ bunches of spinach, washed and dried in a salad spinner (antioxidant)

10–12 slices lean 1% salt bacon

4 hard-boiled eggs, shelled and chopped (antioxidant)

1. In a paper towel-lined microwavable dish, cook bacon slices in microwave on high heat for 12 to 15 minutes until bacon is crisp. Drain fat. Crumble cooked bacon and set aside.
2. Tear spinach into bite-size pieces or halves if necessary and place in a large salad bowl.
3. Sprinkle bacon and eggs on top of spinach.
4. Pour prepared dressing over salad and toss lightly. Chill salad 30 to 45 minutes before serving.

◆ ◆ ◆

Three Bean Salad

(SERVES 6–8)

This tangy bean salad is more suitable for after cancer treatments.

This salad can be stored in an airtight container in the refrigerator for up to 4 days.

½ cup white granulated sugar

½ cup canola oil

½ cup pure apple cider vinegar

1 teaspoon salt

1 × 16 oz/455 mL can cut green beans, drained

1 × 16 oz/455 mL can cut wax beans, drained

1 × 19 oz/540 mL can red kidney beans, drained (antioxidant)

1 small onion, peeled and chopped (antioxidant)

1. Mix together sugar, oil, vinegar and salt in a serving bowl.
2. Stir in three beans and onion until well coated.
3. Cover and refrigerate overnight before serving.

◆ ◆ ◆

Tomato Salad

(SERVES 4)

This healthy salad is fantastic, especially when you use fresh garden tomatoes available during the summer months.

Leftover salad can be stored in a covered container in the refrigerator for up to 3 days.

10 ripe and firm Roma tomatoes, washed and cut into
  wedges (antioxidant)

16 whole black olives with pits

¾ cup Greek Feta cheese, crumbled

2 tablespoons extra virgin olive oil (antioxidant)

2 tablespoons red wine vinegar

¾ teaspoon dried basil leaves

sea salt, to taste

freshly ground black pepper, to taste

1. Place tomato wedges on a large platter.
2. Sprinkle olives and cheese on top.
3. Mix together oil, vinegar, basil, salt and pepper in a small bowl. Drizzle over salad.
4. Chill salad at least 1 hour before serving.

◆ ◆ ◆

Tossed Green Salad

(SERVES 6)

This low-fat salad is a perfect accompaniment to any meal.

Leftover salad can be stored in a covered container in the refrigerator for 2 to 3 days.

1 head green leaf lettuce, washed and dried in a salad spinner

3–4 medium tomatoes, cut into wedges (antioxidant)

½ long English cucumber, cut into wedges

1 bunch radishes, quartered

4 green onions, chopped (antioxidant)

Italian light salad dressing

1. Combine all ingredients in a serving bowl.
2. Toss salad lightly with salad dressing.
3. Cover and chill before serving.

◆ ◆ ◆

Tossed Green Salad with Flax Seed Oil

(SERVES 4)

This was one of Jeff's favourite salad recipes during cancer treatments and post-treatment recovery. It is loaded with antioxidants.

Leftover salad can be stored in a covered container in the refrigerator for up to 3 days.

1 head green leaf lettuce, washed and torn into bite-size pieces

4–5 medium ripe and firm tomatoes, cut into wedges (antioxidant)

2–3 stalks green onions, chopped (antioxidant)

1 medium ripe avocado, pitted, peeled and chunked (antioxidant)

flax seed oil (antioxidant)

1. Combine lettuce, tomatoes and green onions in a large salad bowl. Toss well.
2. Sprinkle avocado chunks on top.
3. Sprinkle 1 teaspoon flax seed oil on each serving of salad.

◆ ◆ ◆

Tossed Salad with Citrus Dressing
(SERVES 4)

The dressing for this salad is both sweet and tangy from the lemon juice, honey and oranges. This salad is loaded with antioxidants.

Leftover salad is best eaten the next day.

> 1 head butter lettuce, washed and torn into bite-size pieces
> 1 small can mandarin orange segments, drained well (antioxidant)
> 1 small red onion, sliced thinly (antioxidant)
> juices of 2 lemons (antioxidant)
> 1 ¾ tablespoons liquid honey
> ¾ tablespoon extra virgin olive oil (antioxidant)
> dash of ground nutmeg
> dash of paprika

1. Combine lettuce, orange and onion in a serving bowl.
2. Mix together lemon juice, honey, oil, nutmeg and paprika in a separate bowl. Pour dressing over salad and toss lightly to coat.
3. Chill before serving.

◆ ◆ ◆

BEEF & PORK

Beef

Pork

Curry and Black Bean Beef

(SERVES 4–6)

This Asian dish is a treat for when you are in the mood for something special. Hot cooked rice is a perfect accompaniment to this meal. However, this somewhat spicy recipe is more suitable between cancer treatments.

Leftovers can be stored in an airtight container in the refrigerator for 2 to 3 days. They can be reheated in the microwave.

1¾–2 lbs beef sirloin steak, cut into 2¼ × ¼-inch strips

1 large egg white

2 tablespoons dry sherry

2 tablespoons dark soy sauce

1½ teaspoons cornstarch

¼ cup extra virgin olive oil (antioxidant)

4–5 green onions, cut into 1¼-inch lengths (antioxidant)

1 medium red bell pepper, seeded and cut into strips (antioxidant)

1½ teaspoons curry powder (antioxidant)

1 tablespoon black bean garlic sauce

2 tablespoons cornstarch mixed with 1 tablespoon water

hot boiled/steamed rice

1. Combine meat, egg, sherry, soy and 1½ teaspoons cornstarch in a bowl. Let stand 40 minutes.

2. Heat oil in a large skillet over medium heat.

3. Cook meat mixture until browned.

4. Add remaining ingredients. Stir until mixture boils and thickens.

◆ ◆ ◆

Karen's Cabbage Rolls

(MAKES 14 EXTRA-LARGE SIZE)

This is our family's favourite recipe. Savoy cabbage is not as gaseous as other cabbages and it is more tender and sweet-tasting. These cabbage rolls were a real treat for Jeff while he was recovering from cancer treatments.

Leftovers can be stored in an airtight container in the refrigerator for 2 to 3 days, and they can be reheated in the microwave. This recipe freezes well in freezer containers for several months.

28 large Savoy cabbage leaves, center vein removed with a knife (antioxidant)
  (or Taiwanese cabbage leaves)

2½ lbs lean ground beef, crumbled

3–3½ cups cooked rice, cooled slightly (antioxidant)

1 medium onion, peeled and chopped (antioxidant)

1 tablespoon Worcestershire sauce

1½ teaspoons salt

½ teaspoon freshly ground black pepper

2 large eggs, beaten (antioxidant)

1 cup skim milk (antioxidant)

3 × 10 oz/284 mL cans condensed tomato soup

3 tablespoons brown sugar

3 tablespoons lemon juice (antioxidant)

1. Boil water in a large pot over high heat.

2. Place cabbage leaves in boiling water for 3 to 4 minutes until limp. Drain well.

3. Combine beef, rice, onion, Worcestershire, salt, pepper, eggs and milk in a large mixing bowl until well mixed.

4. Overlap 2 cabbage leaves, side by side. Spoon ½ cup to ⅔ cup meat mixture on top of leaves. Fold in all sides starting at edge closest to you. Then roll each leaf making sure folded sides are included in roll.

5. Arrange cabbage rolls in two large 9×13×2-inch glass baking dishes.

6. Mix together tomato soup, brown sugar and lemon juice in a bowl. Pour sauce mixture over cabbage rolls.

7. Bake, uncovered and on middle oven rack, in a preheated 350°F oven for 1¼ hours, basting twice with sauce.

◆ ◆ ◆

Karen's Hearty Shepherd's Pie

(SERVES 6–8)

This was Jeff's favourite meat pie. Shepherd's pie is hearty and real comfort food. A green salad rounds out the meal.

Leftover pie is best stored in a covered container in the refrigerator for up to 3 days. It can be reheated in the microwave. This recipe freezes well in freezer containers for several months.

25 g package brown gravy mix

1½ lbs lean ground beef, cooked, crumbled and fat drained

2 × 10 oz/284 mL cans sliced mushrooms, drained well

1 small onion, peeled and chopped (antioxidant)

2–2½ cups frozen mixed vegetables

3 tablespoons ketchup

½ teaspoon dry mustard

salt, to taste

freshly ground black pepper, to taste

6–8 medium russet potatoes, peeled and cut into large chunks (antioxidant)

4 tablespoons margarine

¼–⅓ cup skim milk (antioxidant)

1. Combine gravy mix with 1 cup water in a small saucepan. Cook over medium heat, stirring constantly, until gravy comes to a boil. Then simmer 1 minute.

2. Combine beef, mushrooms, onion, mixed vegetables, ketchup, mustard, salt, pepper and prepared gravy in a large pot. Bring to a boil over medium-high heat. Simmer 5 minutes. Transfer to a 9×13×2-inch glass baking dish.

3. Cook potatoes in boiling water over medium-high heat until fork-tender about 15 to 20 minutes. Drain. Mash potatoes with margarine and milk. Spoon over meat mixture.

4. Bake, on middle oven rack, in a preheated 350°F oven for 25 to 30 minutes.

◆　◆　◆

Glazed Whole Boneless Ham

(SERVES 20–24)

This is an old family-favourite recipe for special occasions.

Leftover ham freezes well when wrapped in aluminum foil and placed in freezer bags.

> **10–12 lb boneless smoked ham, rinsed**
> **whole cloves**
> **¾ cup honey**
> **1½ tablespoons whiskey**

1. Place ham in a foil-lined roasting pan.
2. Insert whole cloves, about two inches apart, all over ham.
3. Combine honey and whiskey in a measuring cup. Mix well. Set aside.
4. Bake ham, on lower oven rack, in a preheated 325°F oven for about 2 hours.
5. Baste ham several times with honey mixture in the last 20 minutes of cooking.

◆ ◆ ◆

Honey and Garlic Pork Spareribs

(SERVES 6)

These were Jeff's favourite pork spareribs. He enjoyed this meal after cancer treatments.

Leftovers can be stored in a covered container in the refrigerator for up to 3 days. They can be reheated in the microwave. This recipe freezes well in freezer containers for up to 3 months.

4½ lbs lean pork spareribs, cut up and fat removed

2 tablespoons medium sherry

2 tablespoons black bean garlic sauce

½ × 112 mL jar of honey garlic sauce

⅔ cup cornstarch

1 small onion, peeled and chunked (or substitute 1 bunch green onions, halved) (antioxidant)

hot boiled/steamed rice (antioxidant)

1. Combine all ingredients, except cornstarch, in a large saucepan.
2. Cook meat mixture over medium heat for 10 minutes. Stir meat with a slotted spoon and cook another 10 minutes.
3. Reduce heat to medium-low. Add cornstarch and cook 17 minutes, stirring occasionally.
4. Serve spareribs with sauce over hot cooked rice.

◆ ◆ ◆

Karen's Curried Pork

(SERVES 6)

The chili paste, five spice powder and coconut milk give this recipe an exotic flavour. This spicy dish is more suitable after cancer treatments.

Leftovers can be stored in a covered container in the refrigerator for up to 3 days. They can be reheated in the microwave.

2½–3 lbs lean pork, cubed ¾-inch

2–3 tablespoons canola oil

½ teaspoon garlic powder

¾ tablespoon ground chili paste

1 medium onion, sliced thinly (antioxidant)

½ cup coconut milk

¼ cup chicken broth

2 tablespoons dry white wine

1 tablespoon curry powder (antioxidant)

½ teaspoon five spice powder

½ teaspoon salt

⅓ teaspoon freshly ground black pepper

3 medium potatoes, cubed ¾-inch (antioxidant)

1 tablespoon cornstarch mixed with 1 teaspoon water

hot boiled/steamed rice (antioxidant)

1. Heat oil in a large pot over medium-high heat.
2. Add meat and cook until browned on all sides.
3. Stir in garlic, chili paste and onion. Cook 3 to 4 minutes.
4. Combine milk, broth, wine, curry, five spice, salt and pepper in a bowl. Add to meat mixture.
5. Add potatoes and bring to a boil. Reduce heat to medium-low, cover and simmer for 25 minutes.
6. Stir in cornstarch mixture until sauce thickens.
7. Serve with hot cooked rice.

• • •

Sweet and Sour Pork

(SERVES 8)

This sweet and tangy recipe is an old family favourite. A tossed green salad completes the meal for dinner.

Leftovers can be stored in a covered container in the refrigerator for up to 3 days. They can be reheated in the microwave. This recipe freezes well in freezer containers for up to 3 months.

2½ lbs lean boneless pork, cubed ¾-inch

3 tablespoons extra virgin olive oil (antioxidant)

½ cup all-purpose flour

¼ cup cornstarch

½ cup cold water

salt, to taste

1 large egg, beaten (antioxidant)

1 × 19 oz/540 mL can unsweetened pineapple chunks, drained and juice reserved (antioxidant)

½ cup brown sugar

½ cup pure white vinegar

1 tablespoon dark soy sauce

4 medium carrots, sliced thinly (antioxidant)

2 tablespoons cornstarch

2 tablespoons cold water

1 large green bell pepper, seeded and chunked (optional) (antioxidant)

hot boiled/steamed rice (antioxidant)

1. Heat oil in a large skillet over medium heat.
2. Combine flour, ¼ cup cornstarch, ½ cup cold water, salt and egg in a bowl. Coat pork cubes in batter.
3. Place prepared pork in skillet and fry 8 to 10 until golden brown. Set aside.
4. Add enough water to reserved pineapple juice to measure 1 cup. Pour into a large saucepan.

5. Stir in brown sugar, vinegar, soy sauce and carrots. Cook over medium heat and bring to a boil about 15 minutes. Then reduce heat to medium-low, cover and simmer about 5 minutes until carrots are crisp-tender.

6. Mix 2 tablespoons cornstarch with 2 tablespoons cold water. Stir into sauce.

7. Add pork and pineapple chunks. Cook over medium heat and bring to a boil, stirring constantly, for 2 to 3 minutes.

8. Serve with hot cooked rice.

◆ ◆ ◆

Teriyaki Pork Loin Chops

(SERVES 4)

Jeff enjoyed this recipe on many occasions with half a potato, a sweet potato and a green salad.

This recipe can be halved, if desired.

2 lean boneless pork loin chops, about ¾ lbs each and ¾-inch thick cut

all-purpose thick teriyaki sauce

1. Place rinsed pork chops in a large non-stick skillet or frying pan.
2. Add teriyaki sauce.
3. Pan fry over medium heat until meat is no longer pink inside. Add water, if necessary, to thin out the sauce.

◆ ◆ ◆

CHICKEN & TURKEY

Asian Chicken and Egg over Rice
(SERVES 4)

This unique dish is ideal for times when you need something different for lunch.

Any leftovers can be stored in an airtight container in the refrigerator overnight. They can be reheated in the microwave the following day.

¾–1 lb skinless and boneless chicken breast, cut into bite-size pieces

6 dried shiitake mushrooms, soaked in hot water 40 minutes, squeezed dry, stems removed and halved (antioxidant)

1 small onion, peeled and sliced thinly (antioxidant)

¼ cup water

4 tablespoons dark soy sauce

3 tablespoons mirin

1 tablespoon white granulated sugar

4 large eggs, beaten (antioxidant)

5 cups hot boiled/steamed rice (antioxidant)

1. Bring water, soy, mirin and sugar in a large skillet to a boil over medium-high heat.
2. Add chicken, mushrooms and onion. Cook over medium heat for 5 to 6 minutes.
3. Pour beaten eggs over chicken.
4. Cook covered, over low heat for 2 to 3 minutes until eggs are set.
5. Place ¼ portion of the cooked rice in each large deep serving bowl.
6. Top with ¼ portion of the chicken and egg mixture.
7. Pour remaining sauce on top.

◆ ◆ ◆

Asian Chicken Casserole

(SERVES 6)

This casserole is aromatic, tender and sweet from the white wine, but it is more suitable between cancer treatments.

Leftover casserole can be stored in an airtight container in the refrigerator for up to 3 days. It can be reheated in the microwave.

2½ lbs skinless and boneless chicken, cut into large pieces

cornstarch

¼ cup extra virgin olive oil (antioxidant)

8 dried shiitake mushrooms, soaked in hot water 40 minutes, squeezed dry and stems removed (antioxidant)

6–8 slices fresh ginger (antioxidant)

1 bunch green onions, cut into 2-inch lengths (antioxidant)

1 clove garlic, peeled and chopped (antioxidant)

1 tablespoon cornstarch, extra

¼ cup chicken broth

⅓ cup dry white wine

1 tablespoon dark soy sauce

½ cup chicken broth, extra

hot boiled/steamed rice (antioxidant)

1. Coat individual chicken pieces with cornstarch.
2. Heat oil and cook chicken in a large saucepan over medium-high heat until golden brown.
3. Add mushrooms, ginger, onions and garlic. Cook 2 minutes.
4. Stir in 1 tablespoon cornstarch, ¼ cup chicken broth, wine and soy sauce. Cook until boiled and thickened.
5. Spoon chicken mixture into a large casserole dish.
6. Pour ½ cup chicken broth evenly on top. Cover with lid.
7. Bake, on middle oven rack, in a preheated 400°F oven for 30 to 40 minutes until chicken is tender.
8. Serve with hot cooked rice.

◆ ◆ ◆

Asian Roast Chicken

(SERVES 8)

This spiced chicken recipe is a nice change from other roast chicken recipes. This recipe can be halved, if desired.

Leftover meat is best stored in an airtight container in the refrigerator for up to 3 days. This recipe freezes well in freezer containers for 2 to 3 months.

2 × 4 lb whole chickens, washed and patted dry
   with paper towels

1¾ tablespoons garlic powder

dash of salt, to taste

freshly ground black pepper, to taste

¼ teaspoon ground nutmeg

¼ teaspoon ground cloves

½ teaspoon ground ginger

½ teaspoon lemon peel

⅓ cup corn syrup

2 tablespoons hoisin sauce

1. Combine all spices and lemon peel together in a small bowl. Rub spice mixture inside cavities and on skin of birds.
2. Place prepared birds in a large foil-lined roasting pan.
3. Mix together corn syrup and hoisin sauce in a measuring cup. Baste chickens in the last 20 minutes of cooking.
4. Bake, on bottom oven rack, in a preheated 350°F oven for 2 to 2¼ hours until done.

◆ ◆ ◆

Caribbean Jerk Chicken

(SERVES 4–5)

This very spicy dish is more suitable after cancer treatments. A tossed green salad makes the perfect accompaniment.

Leftover chicken can be stored in an airtight container in the refrigerator for up to 3 days. It can be reheated in the microwave.

2½ lbs skinless chicken pieces, washed and patted dry
    with paper towels

1 tablespoon ground allspice

¾ tablespoon dried thyme leaves

1 teaspoon ground nutmeg

dash of salt

3–4 green onions, chopped (antioxidant)

2 cloves garlic, peeled and chopped (antioxidant)

2 fresh jalapeño peppers, seeded and chopped

¼ cup freshly squeezed orange juice (antioxidant)

1 tablespoon red wine vinegar

1. Place chicken parts in a shallow glass baking dish.
2. Combine remaining ingredients in a bowl. Pour over chicken and coat both sides of meat.
3. Cover baking dish with plastic wrap and let marinate in refrigerator overnight, turning several times.
4. Remove chicken from marinade. Place on a rack in another shallow baking pan.
5. Bake, on lower oven rack, in a preheated 325°F oven for 45 to 55 minutes until meat is no longer pink inside.

❖ ❖ ❖

Curried Tomato Chicken

(SERVES 4)

This was Jeff's favourite chicken recipe. However, this spicy dish is more suitable after cancer treatments.

Leftover chicken can be stored in an airtight container in the refrigerator for up to 3 days, and it can be reheated in the microwave. This recipe freezes well in freezer containers for 2 to 3 months.

all-purpose cooking spray

1 medium onion, peeled and chopped (antioxidant)

2½–3 tablespoons all-purpose flour

2½ tablespoons curry powder (antioxidant)

dash of garlic powder

1 × 28 oz/796 mL can whole tomatoes, cut up and ½ juice
reserved (antioxidant)

¾ cup natural dark California raisins

juice of 1 lemon (antioxidant)

6 skinless chicken thighs, fat removed

6 skinless chicken drumsticks, fat removed

hot boiled/steamed rice (antioxidant)

1. Spray the bottom of a large saucepan with all-purpose cooking spray.

2. Add onion and cook over medium-low heat for 2 minutes.

3. Stir in flour, curry, garlic and tomatoes. Cook and stir for 3 minutes. Mash tomatoes slightly with a potato masher to thicken sauce.

4. Add raisins and lemon juice. Stir and bring to a boil.

5. Add chicken pieces and cook, covered, over medium-low heat for about 30 minutes until meat is fully cooked. Stir twice during cooking.

6. Serve with hot cooked rice.

◆ ◆ ◆

Fried Chicken

(SERVES 8–10)

This is the best fried chicken recipe, if you don't mind the extra calories. A green salad and mashed potatoes go well with this meal. This recipe can be halved, if desired.

Leftover chicken can be kept in a covered container in the refrigerator for up to 3 days. Cold cooked chicken is still tasty the next day. It can be reheated in the oven, too.

6 lbs mixed chicken pieces (breasts, thighs and drumsticks)
⅔ cup all-purpose flour
1¼ tablespoons paprika
1 tablespoon salt
½ teaspoon freshly ground black pepper
canola oil

1. Combine flour, paprika, salt and pepper in a mixing bowl.
2. Coat chicken parts in flour mixture.
3. Deep fry chicken in hot oil, about 375°F, for 12 to 15 minutes until both sides are cooked and browned.
4. Transfer chicken to paper-towel lined baking sheets to drain fat.

◆ ◆ ◆

Hawaiian Chicken

(SERVES 4–6)

This is a sweet and tangy tropical dish. A tossed green salad is a perfect accompaniment to this meal.

Leftovers can be stored in an airtight container in the refrigerator for up to 3 days. They can be reheated in the microwave.

all-purpose cooking spray

4½ lbs skinless chicken thighs and drumsticks

dash of salt

dash of freshly ground black pepper

1 × 19 oz/540 mL can unsweetened pineapple chunks, drained and juice reserved (antioxidant)

⅔ cup water

½ cup pure white vinegar

½ cup golden yellow sugar

2 tablespoons dark soy sauce

1 teaspoon salt

3½ tablespoons cornstarch

1 medium green bell pepper, seeded and cut into chunks (optional) (antioxidant)

hot boiled/steamed rice (antioxidant)

1. Spray the bottom of a large skillet or frying pan with all-purpose cooking spray.
2. Brown chicken on both sides over medium heat for 10 to 12 minutes.
3. Sprinkle salt and pepper over chicken.
4. Transfer chicken to a large casserole dish.
5. Add remaining ingredients, except green pepper and pineapple, to skillet. Cook and stir over medium-high heat until mixture boils and thickens (about 4 to 5 minutes).
6. Stir in pineapple and green pepper. Pour over chicken.
7. Cover casserole dish with aluminum foil.
8. Bake, on lower oven rack, in a preheated 350°F oven for about 1½ hours until tender.
9. Serve with hot cooked rice.

◆ ◆ ◆

Honey Curry Chicken

(SERVES 8–10)

This is one of our favourite sweet curry recipes.

Leftovers can be stored in an airtight container in the refrigerator for up to 3 days. It can be reheated in the microwave. This recipe freezes well in freezer containers for up to 3 months.

18–20 chicken pieces (thighs and drumsticks)

⅓ cup margarine, melted

¾ cup honey

½ cup prepared mustard

4 tablespoons curry powder (antioxidant)

2 × 10 oz/284 mL cans sliced mushrooms, juice of one can reserved

hot boiled/steamed rice (antioxidant)

1. Brown chicken on both sides in a large saucepan over medium-high heat.
2. Transfer chicken to a large casserole dish.
3. Mix together remaining ingredients in a bowl and pour over chicken.
4. Bake, on lower oven rack, in a preheated 325°F oven for 1¼ to 1½ hours. Turn chicken occasionally until coated in sauce.
5. Serve with hot cooked rice.

◆ ◆ ◆

Honey Garlic Chicken

(SERVES 6)

This is a quick and simple dish that can be reheated in the microwave the next day.

3–3½ lbs skinless and boneless chicken, cut up into bite-size chunks
(mixed white and dark meat preferred)

fresh ginger root, sliced thinly (antioxidant)

1 bunch green onions, sliced diagonally into 2-inch lengths (antioxidant)

⅓ × 225 mL jar of honey garlic sauce

1½ tablespoons black bean garlic sauce

⅓–½ cup cornstarch

hot boiled/steamed rice (antioxidant)

1. Combine all ingredients, except cornstarch, in a large saucepan.
2. Cook, covered, over medium-high heat for 15 minutes.
3. Add cornstarch and stir well.
4. Reduce heat to medium and cook, covered, another 10 minutes until tender.
5. Serve with hot cooked rice.

◆ ◆ ◆

Oven-Baked Spiced Chicken

(SERVES 5–6)

This chicken is crisp on the outside and juicy and tender on the inside. A baked potato or sweet potato and a green salad are the perfect accompaniments to this meal.

This spicy recipe is more suitable for after cancer treatments.

Leftover chicken can be stored in a covered container in the refrigerator for 2 to 3 days. It is just as tasty the next day when reheated in the microwave.

4 lb whole chicken, skin removed and halved

extra virgin olive oil (antioxidant)

1¼ tablespoons paprika

1 teaspoon freshly ground black pepper

dash of salt

½ teaspoon dried oregano leaves

½ teaspoon dry mustard

pinch of cayenne pepper

1. Place chicken halves, skin side up, on a large foil-lined baking sheet.
2. Brush oil on top of chicken.
3. Combine remaining ingredients in a bowl. Sprinkle evenly over chicken.
4. Let stand at room temperature for 30 minutes.
5. Bake, on middle oven rack, in a preheated 375°F oven for about 1 hour until fully cooked.

◆ ◆ ◆

Spanish Paella

(SERVES 6)

This simple and elegant one-pan meal is full of antioxidants.

Leftovers can be stored in a covered container in the refrigerator for 2 days. They can be reheated in the microwave the next day.

all-purpose cooking spray

½ lb cooked shrimp, rinsed and drained well

1½ lbs chicken thighs and drumsticks, washed and pat dry
    with paper towels

1 medium onion, peeled and chopped (antioxidant)

dash of garlic powder

1 × 14½ oz/412 mL can chicken broth

1 × 7½ oz can whole tomatoes, cut up in juices (antioxidant)

⅓ teaspoon ground saffron

dash of hot chili powder

1 cup long grain rice (antioxidant)

1 medium red bell pepper, seeded and cut into chunks (antioxidant)

1¼ cups frozen peas

1. Spray the bottom of a large skillet with all-purpose cooking spray.

2. Cook onion and garlic over medium heat until tender.

3. Add chicken, broth, undrained tomatoes, saffron and chili powder. Bring to a boil and then reduce heat to medium-low. Simmer, covered, for 15 minutes.

4. Stir in rice and simmer, covered, for another 15 minutes.

5. Add shrimp, red pepper and peas. Cook 5 to 7 minutes more.

◆ ◆ ◆

Spicy Almond Chicken

(SERVES 8–10)

This is one of our favourite spicy chicken recipes for after cancer treatments. It is loaded with antioxidants, such as the almonds that give this dish an added crunch. A tossed green salad is the perfect accompaniment to this dish.

Leftovers can be stored in a covered container in the refrigerator for 2 to 3 days. They can be reheated in the microwave.

½ cup ketchup (or substitute ½ cup tomato sauce + ¼ cup sugar +
    1 tablespoon vinegar) (antioxidant)

3½ tablespoons dark soy sauce

¼ teaspoon salt

2½ tablespoons Worcestershire sauce

3 tablespoons white granulated sugar

½ cup chicken broth

2 whole skinless and boneless chicken breasts, cut into bite-size chunks

4½ tablespoons cornstarch

dash of salt

4 tablespoons extra virgin olive oil (antioxidant)

16 thin slices fresh ginger (antioxidant)

1 clove garlic, peeled and chopped (antioxidant)

dash of sesame oil

1 medium onion, peeled and sliced thinly (antioxidant)

1 jalapeño pepper, seeded and chopped

1 large red bell pepper, seeded and cut into strips (antioxidant)

2 large carrots, sliced thinly on diagonal (antioxidant)

2⅓ cups frozen cut green beans

1½ cups natural whole almonds (antioxidant)

hot boiled/steamed rice (antioxidant)

1. Mix together ketchup, soy sauce, salt, Worcestershire, sugar and chicken broth in a bowl. Set aside.
2. Combine chicken, cornstarch and salt in another bowl. Set aside.

3. Heat olive oil in a large non-stick skillet over medium heat.

4. Cook ginger, garlic, sesame oil, onion and jalapeño for 4 minutes.

5. Add chicken mixture and cook, covered, over medium-low heat for 10 minutes until almost cooked.

6. Stir in red pepper, carrots and beans. Cook, covered, for 4 minutes.

7. Add sauce mixture and cook, covered, over medium-high heat for 4 to 5 minutes until sauce comes to a boil.

8. Remove from heat and stir in almonds.

9. Serve with hot cooked rice.

◆ ◆ ◆

Teriyaki Chicken Breast Fajitas

(SERVES 4)

This easy-to-make recipe comes in handy for lunch or dinner when you have a busy schedule and limited time to cook. Jeff enjoyed this meal after his medical appointments. It is full of antioxidants.

Leftover chicken can be reheated in the microwave the next day.

  2 whole skinless and boneless chicken breasts, cut across the grain and into long strips

  ⅓–½ cup all-purpose thick teriyaki sauce

  1 medium green bell pepper, seeded and cut into strips (antioxidant)

  1 medium red onion, peeled and sliced thinly (antioxidant)

  1 large ripe avocado, pitted, peeled and sliced lengthwise into 8s (antioxidant)

  2–3 medium ripe tomatoes, seeded and chopped (antioxidant)

  8 small (about 6-inch diameter) soft flour tortillas

1. Cook chicken strips with teriyaki sauce in a large non-stick skillet over medium-high heat for 10 minutes until meat is no longer pink inside.
2. Stir in pepper and onion strips. Cook another 5 minutes.
3. Spoon chicken mixture on center of each tortilla.
4. Top with 2 avocado slices and chopped tomatoes.
5. Fold both sides over center of tortilla with edges overlapping.

◆ ◆ ◆

Easy-To-Make Turkey Casserole

(SERVES 6–7)

This quick and simple recipe comes in handy when you need to prepare a hearty and filling meal. A tossed green salad is the perfect accompaniment to this casserole.

Leftover casserole is best stored in a covered container in the refrigerator for 2 days. It can be reheated in the microwave. This recipe freezes well in freezer containers for up to 3 months.

5 tablespoons margarine

⅓ cup all-purpose flour

½ teaspoon dried marjoram leaves

freshly ground black pepper, to taste

1 cup skim milk (antioxidant)

1 × 10 oz/284 mL can chicken broth

3½ cups cooked turkey breast, cubed ½-inch

5–6 cups frozen mixed vegetables, partially thawed

1. Melt margarine in a large saucepan over medium heat.
2. Stir in flour, marjoram and pepper. Cook, stirring, until mixture is smooth and bubbly.
3. Add milk and broth. Cook and stir until mixture boils and thickens.
4. Stir in turkey and vegetables. Cook, stirring occasionally, about 15 minutes until vegetables are tender. Spoon mixture into casserole dish and serve immediately.

◆ ◆ ◆

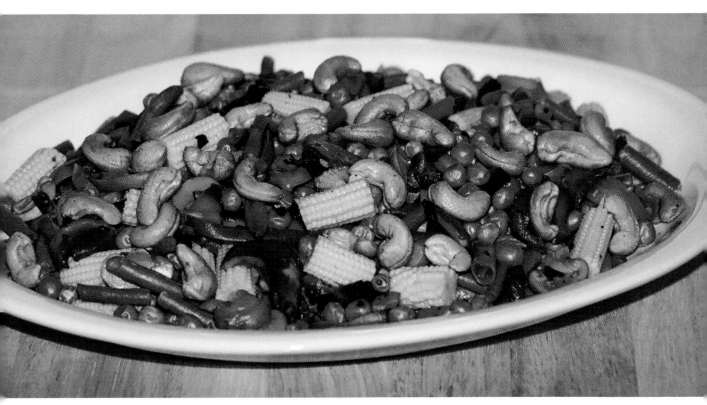

Mixed Vegetables with Cashew Nuts
Recipe on Page 232

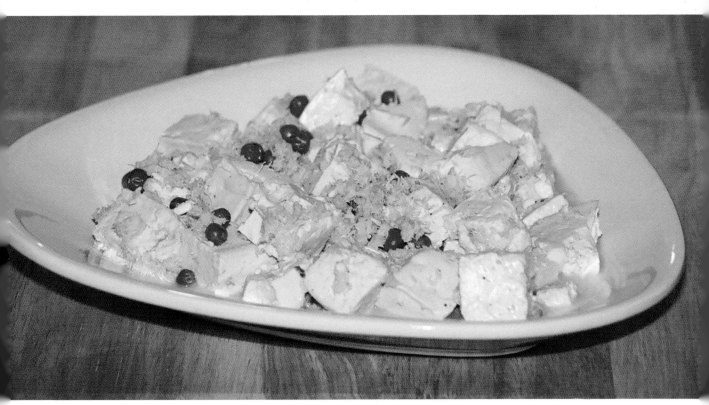

Tofu with Crabmeat
Recipe on Page 201

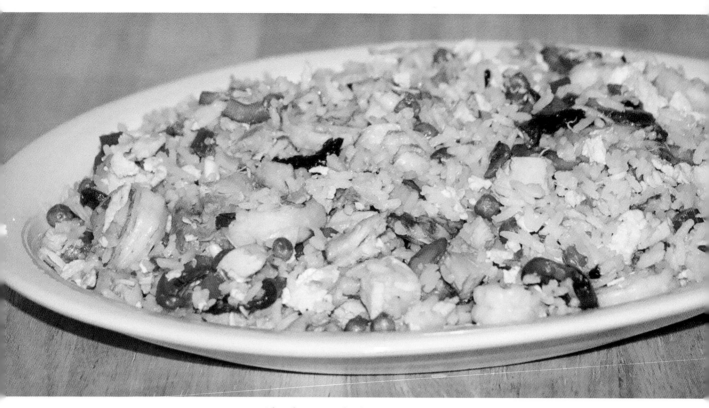

Chicken and Shrimp Fried Rice

Recipe on Page 219

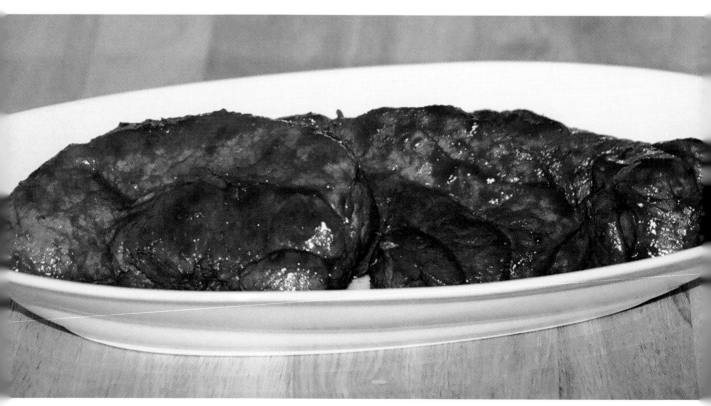

Teriyaki Pork Loin Chops

Recipe on Page 176

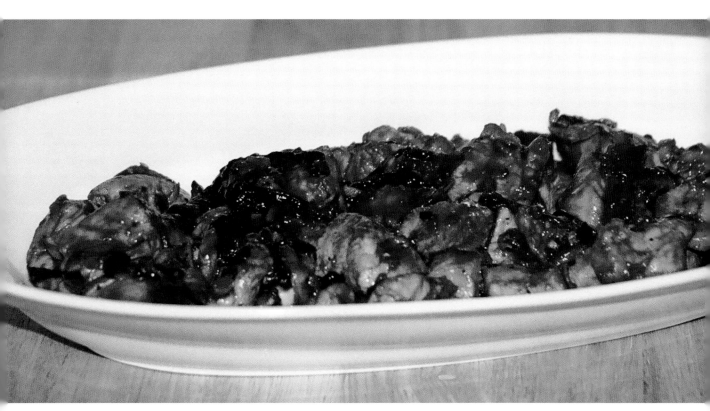

Honey Garlic Chicken
Recipe on Page 186

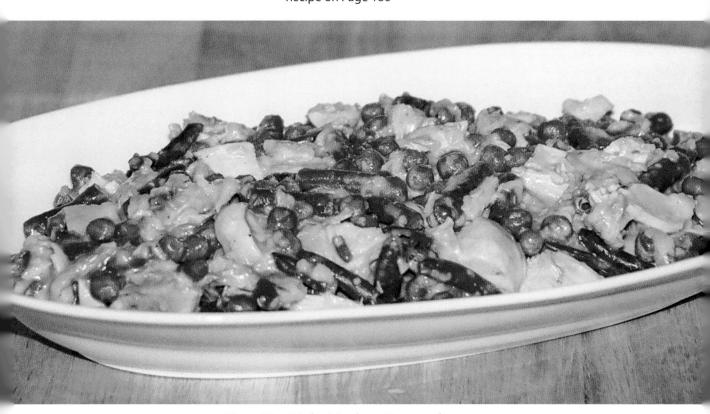

Easy-To-Make Turkey Casserole
Recipe on Page 192

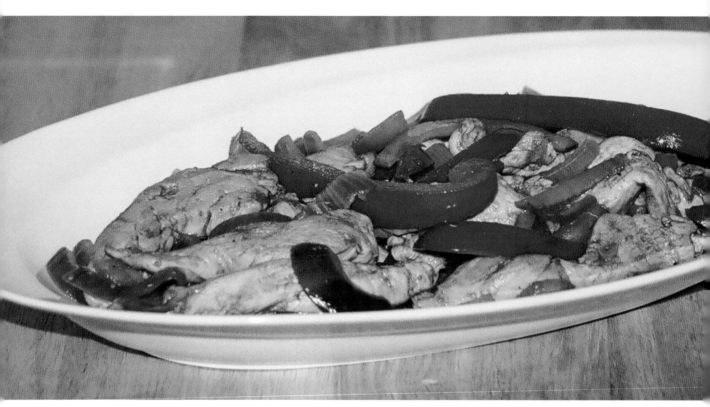

Teriyaki Chicken Breast Fajitas
Recipe on Page 191

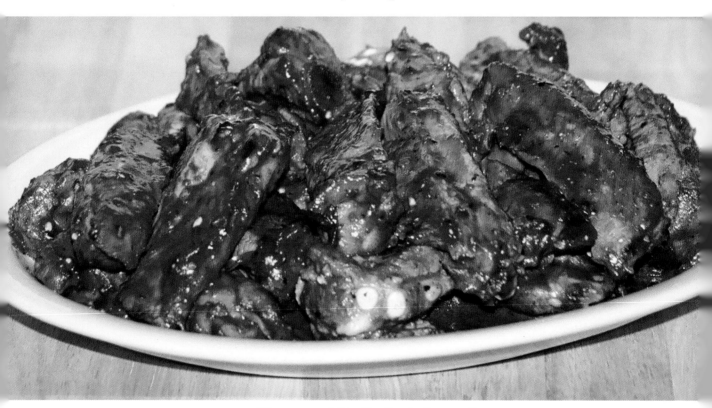

Honey and Garlic Pork Spareribs
Recipe on Page 172

Roast Honey and Spice Turkey

(SERVES 12–16)

This spiced turkey with exotic flavours has been our favourite recipe for years. Jeff enjoyed a turkey drumstick or thigh with half a baked potato, a sweet potato and a green salad.

Leftover turkey is best stored in a covered container in the refrigerator for up to 3 days. It can be reheated in the microwave or enjoyed in a cold turkey breast sandwich. This recipe freezes well for several months when wrapped in aluminum foil and placed in freezer bags.

8–10 lb turkey, halved, washed and dried with paper towels

2 tablespoons salt

2 tablespoons freshly ground black pepper

1 tablespoon ground ginger

1 teaspoon five spice powder

½ cup corn syrup

4 tablespoons dark soy sauce

1. Combine salt, pepper, ginger and five spice powder in a bowl. Sprinkle mixture on the cavity of each half of turkey. Rub remaining spice mixture on skin of turkey.

2. Place turkey halves on a rack in a large deep roasting pan.

3. Bake, covered and on bottom rack, in a preheated 350°F oven for up to 2½ hours.

4. Combine corn syrup and soy sauce in a measuring cup. Baste turkey with soy mixture in the last 20 to 25 minutes of cooking time. Remove aluminum foil.

◆ ◆ ◆

Spanish Turkey and Rice

(SERVES 4)

This simple recipe is healthy and low in fat. The green olives add a Mediterranean flavour.

Any leftovers can be reheated in the microwave the following day.

all-purpose cooking spray

¾ lb turkey breast, cut into bite-size chunks

1 small onion, peeled and chopped (antioxidant)

⅓ cup pitted green olives, chopped

1½ teaspoons dried oregano leaves

dash of garlic powder

freshly ground black pepper, to taste

1 cup long grain rice, rinsed and drained (antioxidant)

1 × 14½ oz/412 mL can chicken broth

¼ cup water

2 medium tomatoes, chopped (antioxidant)

1 cup frozen peas

1. Spray the bottom of a large skillet with all-purpose cooking spray.
2. Cook turkey over medium-high heat for 4 to 5 minutes until browned. Set aside.
3. Add onion, olives, oregano, garlic and pepper to skillet. Cook over medium heat 3 to 4 minutes.
4. Stir in turkey, rice, broth and water. Bring to a boil over medium heat. Then reduce heat to medium-low and simmer, covered, about 15 minutes until liquid is absorbed and rice is tender.
5. Stir in tomatoes and peas. Heat through for 2 to 3 minutes more.

◆ ◆ ◆

SEAFOOD & TOFU

Braised Shrimp with Vegetables

(SERVES 4)

This is a quick and light meal.

Leftovers can be stored in a covered container in the refrigerator. They can be reheated in the microwave the next day.

1 tablespoon extra virgin olive oil (antioxidant)

1 lb large shrimp, shelled and deveined

½ lb broccoli flowerets, cut into bite-size pieces (antioxidant)

1 × 10 oz/284 mL can whole mushrooms, drained well

⅓–½ cup chicken broth

1½ teaspoons cornstarch

1 teaspoon oyster sauce

pinch of white granulated sugar

1 teaspoon fresh ginger, chopped (antioxidant)

freshly ground black pepper, to taste

hot boiled/steamed rice (antioxidant)

1. Heat oil in a large skillet over medium-high heat.
2. Add shrimp and stir-fry about 3 minutes until pink.
3. Add broccoli and stir-fry 1 minute.
4. Add mushrooms and stir-fry 1 minute.
5. Combine remaining ingredients in a mixing bowl. Stir well. Pour over shrimp and vegetables. Cook and stir until sauce boils and thickens, about 2 minutes.
6. Serve with hot cooked rice.

◆ ◆ ◆

Prawns with Vegetables

(SERVES 4)

This simple-to-make meal goes well with a tossed green salad.

Leftovers can be kept in a covered container in the refrigerator. They can be reheated in the microwave the next day.

1¼ lbs cooked prawns, rinsed and drained

¾ lb broccoli flowerets, cut up (antioxidant)

1 × 10 oz/284 mL can whole mushrooms, drained well

⅓ cup chicken broth

1 tablespoon cornstarch mixed with 1 teaspoon water

1 tablespoon oyster sauce

4 thin slices fresh ginger (antioxidant)

hot boiled/steamed rice (antioxidant)

1. Combine all ingredients in a large skillet.
2. Bring to a boil over medium-high heat, stirring constantly. Cook 3 to 4 minutes more.
3. Serve with hot cooked rice.

◆ ◆ ◆

Steamed Whole Tilapia Fish
(SERVES 3–4)

Tilapia is a sweet and delicate white fish. Baked squash, baked potatoes and steamed broccoli go well with this meal. This fish is best eaten on the same day it is prepared.

2 lb whole Tilapia fish with head and tail, gutted, cleaned and scaled

½ teaspoon salt

½ teaspoon white pepper

dash of garlic powder

small fresh ginger root, sliced thinly (antioxidant)

3 green onions, cut into 2-inch lengths (antioxidant)

1 tablespoon sesame oil (or canola oil)

2 tablespoons soy sauce

1. Slash fish on both sides diagonally with a sharp knife. Make three cuts on each side.
2. Stuff inside of fish with salt, pepper, garlic, ginger and onions. Rub remaining mixture into cuts on both sides.
3. Place prepared fish in a large shallow dish.
4. Sprinkle sesame oil and soy sauce over fish.
5. Place dish in a large saucepan.
6. Steam fish over medium-high heat for 25 to 30 minutes until fully cooked.

◆ ◆ ◆

Asian Curried Tofu

(SERVES 4)

This spicy meal is more suitable for after cancer treatments.

Leftovers can be kept in a covered container in the refrigerator. They can be reheated in the microwave the next day.

1 tablespoon extra virgin olive oil (antioxidant) (or canola oil)

2–3 green onions, chopped (antioxidant)

1 tablespoon fresh ginger, chopped (antioxidant)

dash of garlic powder

½ lb/225 g lean ground beef, crumbled

½ teaspoon curry powder (antioxidant)

dash of chili powder

2 tablespoons dark soy sauce

½ cup chicken broth (or beef broth)

1 tablespoon cornstarch mixed with 1 teaspoon water

700 g package smooth or traditional tofu, drained well and cut into
   ½-inch cubes (antioxidant)

¼ cup cooked green peas

hot boiled/steamed rice (antioxidant)

1. Heat oil in a large skillet over high heat.
2. Stir-fry onions, ginger and garlic for 2 minutes.
3. Add beef and stir-fry over medium heat until meat is no longer pink inside.
4. Add curry, chili powder, soy sauce and broth. Bring to a boil.
5. Add cornstarch mixture and stir until combined.
6. Add tofu, stir and simmer over low heat until thickened.
7. Stir in cooked peas.
8. Serve with hot cooked rice.

◆ ◆ ◆

Asian Spicy Tofu

(SERVES 4)

This spicy dish is more suitable for after cancer treatments.

Leftovers can be kept in a covered container in the refrigerator. They can be reheated in the microwave the next day.

1 tablespoon extra virgin olive oil (antioxidant) (or canola oil)

2–3 green onions, chopped (antioxidant)

1 tablespoon fresh ginger, chopped (antioxidant)

dash of garlic powder

¾ teaspoon dried crushed red chilies

½ lb/225 g lean ground beef, crumbled

2 tablespoons ketchup

2 tablespoons dark soy sauce

½ cup chicken broth (or beef broth)

1 tablespoon cornstarch mixed with 1 teaspoon water

700 g package smooth or traditional tofu, drained well and cut into
    ½-inch cubes (antioxidant)

¼ cup cooked green peas

hot boiled/steamed rice (antioxidant)

1. Heat oil in a large skillet over high heat.
2. Stir-fry onions, ginger, garlic and chilies for 2 minutes.
3. Add beef and stir-fry over medium heat until meat is no longer pink inside.
4. Add ketchup, soy sauce and broth. Bring to a boil.
5. Add cornstarch mixture and stir until combined.
6. Add tofu, stir and simmer over low heat until thickened.
7. Stir in cooked peas.
8. Serve with hot cooked rice.

◆ ◆ ◆

Tofu with Crabmeat

(SERVES 4)

The crabmeat in this recipe gives this dish a different flavour and texture.

Leftovers can be kept in a covered container in the refrigerator. They can be reheated in the microwave the next day.

¾ tablespoon extra virgin olive oil (antioxidant) (or canola oil)

dash of ground ginger

1 × 4 oz/120 g can crabmeat, drained well

dash of salt

1 teaspoon white granulated sugar

½–⅔ cup chicken broth

1 tablespoon cornstarch

sprinkle of dry white wine

dash of freshly ground black pepper

¼ cup cooked green peas

700 g package firm tofu, drained well and cut into
      ¾-inch cubes (antioxidant)

hot boiled/steamed rice (antioxidant)

1. Heat oil with ginger in a large skillet over medium-high heat.
2. Add crabmeat and stir for a few minutes until cooked.
3. Stir in remaining ingredients and cook until thickened.
4. Serve with hot cooked rice.

◆　◆　◆

Tofu with Mushrooms and Peas

(SERVES 4–5)

This vegetarian recipe is healthy and low in fat.

Leftovers can be kept in a covered container in the refrigerator. They can be reheated in the microwave the next day.

1 tablespoon extra virgin olive oil (antioxidant)

dash of ground ginger

1 × 10 oz/284 mL can whole mushrooms, drained well

700 g package firm tofu, drained and cut into 1-inch cubes (antioxidant)

1¼ cups frozen green peas, partially thawed

3 tablespoons oyster sauce

⅓–½ cup chicken broth

dash of dry sherry (optional)

freshly ground black pepper, to taste

2 tablespoons cornstarch mixed with 1 tablespoon water

hot boiled/steamed rice (antioxidant)

1. Heat oil in a large skillet over medium heat.
2. Stir-fry ginger and mushrooms for 3 to 4 minutes.
3. Add remaining ingredients, except cornstarch mixture, and heat until hot.
4. Stir in cornstarch mixture and cook until thickened.
5. Serve with hot cooked rice.

◆ ◆ ◆

Tofu with Oyster Sauce

(SERVES 4)

This low-fat recipe is suitable for those days when you wish to have a meatless meal.

Leftovers can be kept in a covered container in the refrigerator. They can be reheated in the microwave the next day.

all-purpose cooking spray

350 g package firm tofu, drained and cut into 1-inch cubes (antioxidant)

2–3 celery stalks, sliced diagonally ½-inch (antioxidant)

4 green onions, cut into 1-inch lengths (antioxidant)

1 × 10 oz/284 mL can sliced mushrooms, drained well

2 tablespoons cornstarch mixed with 1 tablespoon water

3 tablespoons oyster sauce

hot boiled/steamed rice (antioxidant)

1. Spray the bottom of a large skillet with all-purpose cooking spray.
2. Stir-fry celery, onions and mushrooms over medium-high heat for a few minutes.
3. Add tofu, cornstarch mixture and oyster sauce. Stir gently. Cook, stirring occasionally, until sauce boils.
4. Serve with hot cooked rice.

◆ ◆ ◆

Tofu with Pork

(SERVES 4–5)

This Asian dish goes well with hot cooked rice.

Leftovers can be kept in a covered container in the refrigerator. They can be reheated in the microwave the next day.

½ lb sliced Chinese barbecued pork

1 tablespoon oyster sauce

dash of dark soy sauce

1 teaspoon Chinese bean sauce

700 g package traditional smooth tofu, drained and cut into
¾-inch cubes (antioxidant)

2–3 green onions, cut into 1½-inch lengths (antioxidant)

2 tablespoons cornstarch mixed with 1 teaspoon water

hot boiled/steamed rice (antioxidant)

1. Cook pork with sauces in a medium saucepan over medium heat for 4 to 5 minutes.

2. Stir in tofu, onions and cornstarch mixture. Cook a few minutes more until heated through.

3. Serve with hot cooked rice.

♦ ♦ ♦

Tofu with Vegetables
(SERVES 2)

This recipe is healthy, low-fat and perfect for those who prefer a vegetarian meal.

Leftovers can be reheated in the microwave the next day.

1 tablespoon canola oil

3 celery stalks, sliced diagonally ½-inch thick (antioxidant)

6 green onions, sliced diagonally into 1½-inch lengths (antioxidant)

½ cup shiitake mushrooms, soaked in boiling water 40 minutes, squeezed dry, stems removed and sliced thinly (antioxidant)

1½ tablespoons cornstarch mixed with ⅓ cup water

2 tablespoons oyster sauce

1 tablespoon soy sauce

1 tablespoon dry sherry (optional)

8 oz/250 g firm tofu, cut into 1-inch cubes (antioxidant)

hot boiled/steamed rice (antioxidant)

1. Heat oil in a large saucepan over medium heat.
2. Add vegetables and sauté 3 to 4 minutes.
3. Stir in remaining ingredients and cook until sauce boils.
4. Serve with hot cooked rice.

◆ ◆ ◆

PASTA & RICE

Cheesy Rigatoni and Broccoli Casserole

(SERVES 6–8)

This casserole was one of Jeff's favourite pasta recipes. It is not low in calories, so it is best served when weight loss occurs due to cancer treatments.

Leftover casserole is best kept in a covered container in the refrigerator for 2 days. It can be reheated in the microwave.

2½–2¾ cups rigatoni (tube-shaped pasta) shells, cooked according to
   package directions and drained well

2–2½ cups broccoli crowns, cut up (antioxidant)

all-purpose cooking spray

1 tablespoon all-purpose flour

dash of salt

1¼ cups Creamo (or half and half)

1 cup Swiss cheese, grated (light preferred)

1 cup light medium Cheddar cheese, grated

½ cup Parmesan cheese, grated

fine bread crumbs

1. Combine cooked pasta and broccoli in a large mixing bowl. Let stand for 5 minutes. Set aside.
2. Spray the bottom of a large saucepan with all-purpose cooking spray.
3. Cook and stir flour and salt over medium heat for 1 minute.
4. Add Creamo and cook until mixture thickens, stirring constantly. Remove from heat.
5. Add three cheeses and stir until melted.
6. Stir in pasta and broccoli until well mixed.
7. Pour mixture into a 2-quart or 8-inch square glass baking dish.
8. Sprinkle bread crumbs on top.
9. Bake, on middle oven rack, in a preheated 350°F oven for 30 to 40 minutes until bubbly and golden brown.

◆ ◆ ◆

Ham and Cheese Pasta Salad

(SERVES 6–8)

This pasta salad recipe is perfect for those hot summer days when you do not want to spend a lot of time in the kitchen.

Leftover salad can be kept in a covered container in the refrigerator for up to 3 days.

2¼–2½ cups rotini twists (corkscrew pasta), cooked according to package directions, rinsed and drained well

2 cups Black Forest ham, cubed ½-inch

1½–1¾ cups light medium Cheddar cheese, cubed ½-inch

2–3 medium tomatoes, cut into bite-size chunks (antioxidant)

1 medium green bell pepper, cut into bite-size chunks (antioxidant)

⅔–¾ cup light Italian dressing

1. Mix together all ingredients in a large salad bowl until well blended.
2. Cover and refrigerate at least 2 to 3 hours before serving.

◆ ◆ ◆

Homemade Spaghetti Sauce

(SERVES 10–12)

This pasta sauce is one of our oldest family-favourite recipes. It is also loaded with antioxidants from the tomatoes and peppers.

Leftovers can be kept in a covered container in the refrigerator for up to 3 days. This recipe freezes well in freezer containers for several months.

4–4½ lbs lean ground beef

2 × 14 oz/398 mL cans all-purpose tomato sauce (antioxidant)

3 × 5½ oz/156 mL cans tomato paste (antioxidant)

1 × 28 oz/796 mL can whole tomatoes, cut up with juices (antioxidant)

2½ large onions, peeled and chopped (antioxidant)

2 medium red bell peppers, seeded and chopped (antioxidant)

1 medium green bell pepper, seeded and chopped (antioxidant)

2 lbs fresh white mushrooms, washed and sliced thinly

salt, to taste

freshly ground black pepper, to taste

cooked spaghetti

freshly grated Parmesan cheese

1. Crumble ground beef in a large pot with a wooden spoon. Brown meat over medium-high heat for 15 to 18 minutes until it is no longer pink inside. Drain fat.
2. Add remaining ingredients and stir well.
3. Cook, covered, for 1¼ to 1½ hours over medium-low heat. Stir occasionally.
4. Serve with cooked spaghetti noodles.
5. Sprinkle cheese on top.

◆ ◆ ◆

Macaroni and Cheese

(SERVES 6–8)

Jeff enjoyed this classic dish at lunch with a green salad and a whole wheat bun.

Leftovers can be kept in a covered container in the refrigerator for 2 days. They can be reheated in the microwave. This recipe freezes well in freezer containers for up to 2 months.

> **2 cups macaroni shells, cooked about 6 minutes in boiling water and drained**
> **2 tablespoons margarine**
> **¼ cup all-purpose flour**
> **2½ cups skim milk** (antioxidant)
> **1 tablespoon Dijon mustard**
> **1 teaspoon salt**
> **dash of freshly ground black pepper**
> **2 cups light medium Cheddar cheese, grated**

1. Whisk together margarine and flour in a large saucepan over medium heat.
2. Add milk, mustard, salt and pepper. Whisk again to remove all lumps. Stir until boiled.
3. Stir in 1½ cups cheese until melted.
4. Add cooked pasta and stir until well mixed.
5. Pour pasta mixture into an 8-inch square glass baking dish.
6. Sprinkle remaining ½ cup cheese on top.
7. Broil in oven on top rack for about 6 minutes until cheese melts.

◆ ◆ ◆

Mixed Seafood Fettuccine
(SERVES 8)

This has been one of our favourite pasta recipes over the years. A tossed green salad is the perfect accompaniment to this seafood dish.

This recipe can be halved, if desired. Leftovers can be reheated in the microwave the next day.

1 ½ lbs prawns, shelled and rinsed

3–4 garlic cloves, peeled and sliced (antioxidant)

¾ lb fettuccine noodles, cooked according to package directions
    and drained

1 × 142 g can clams, drained and ½ can juice reserved

⅓ cup dry white wine

1 cup whipping cream

1 tablespoon margarine

¾ cup Parmesan cheese, grated

salt, to taste

freshly ground black pepper, to taste

1. Marinate prawns in garlic slices for at least 2 hours in a covered bowl.
2. Cook clams, clam juice and wine in a large saucepan over medium heat for 5 minutes.
3. Add whipping cream and heat for 5 minutes.
4. Stir in prawns and cook 3 minutes.
5. Add pasta, margarine, Parmesan, salt and pepper. Cook and stir until thickened.

◆ ◆ ◆

Pasta Meat Sauce

(SERVES 6–8)

This is another recipe that has been an old family favourite over the years. This meaty sauce is full of antioxidants.

Leftover sauce can be kept in a covered container in the refrigerator for up to 3 days. It can be reheated in the microwave. This recipe freezes well in freezer containers for several months.

2¼ lbs lean ground beef

1 large onion, peeled and chopped (antioxidant)

2 × 10 oz/284 mL cans sliced mushrooms, drained

1 × 28 oz/796 mL can whole tomatoes, cut up in juices (antioxidant)

2 × 5½ oz/156 mL cans pure tomato paste (antioxidant)

1 × 24 oz/680 mL can all-purpose tomato sauce (antioxidant)

salt, to taste

freshly ground black pepper, to taste

¾ teaspoon garlic powder

1 teaspoon dried oregano leaves

¾ teaspoon dried basil leaves

1 medium green bell pepper, seeded and chopped (optional) (antioxidant)

1. Crumble ground beef in a large pot with a wooden spoon. Cook over medium-high heat for 13 to 15 minutes until meat is no longer pink inside. Drain fat.

2. Stir in remaining ingredients until well blended. Cook another 45 to 50 minutes.

3. Serve with your favourite cooked pasta shells. Sprinkle grated Parmesan cheese on top, if desired.

◆ ◆ ◆

Seafood Fettuccine Alfredo

(SERVES 8)

This is our favourite pasta recipe, even with the extra calories. Jeff always enjoyed a second serving, especially after cancer treatments.

This recipe can be halved, if desired.

Leftovers can be stored in a covered container in the refrigerator. They can be reheated in the microwave the next day.

- 1 lb/450 g fettuccine noodles, cooked according to package directions and drained
- ¼ cup margarine
- 1 cup/250 mL whipping cream
- ¾ cup Parmesan cheese, grated
- 2 × 7½ oz/213 g cans sockeye salmon, juices drained (antioxidant)
- 1 lb/450 g cooked prawns

1. Melt margarine with whipping cream and Parmesan cheese in a large saucepan over medium-low heat.
2. Add salmon and prawns. Cook 2 to 3 minutes.
3. Stir in cooked noodles and mix well. Cook about 5 minutes more.

◆ ◆ ◆

Seafood Lasagne

(SERVES 6–8)

This is the best seafood lasagne you will ever taste, but it is not low in calories.

Leftover lasagne can be kept in a covered container in the refrigerator for 1 to 2 days. It can be reheated in the microwave the next day.

10–12 lasagne noodles, cooked according to package directions and drained well

2 tablespoons margarine

1 medium onion, peeled and chopped (antioxidant)

8 oz package light cream cheese

1½ cups light creamed cottage cheese

2 large eggs, beaten (antioxidant)

¾ tablespoon dried basil leaves

salt, to taste

freshly ground black pepper, to taste

2 × 10 oz/284 mL cans condensed cream of mushroom soup

⅓ cup skim milk (antioxidant)

⅓ cup dry white wine

1 × 120 g can crabmeat, drained well

1¼ lbs cooked shrimp

¼ cup Parmesan cheese, grated

¾ cup aged Cheddar cheese, shredded

1. Melt margarine in a large saucepan over medium heat.
2. Stir in chopped onions and cook until tender.
3. Mix in remaining ingredients except cheeses.
4. Layer ½ each of the cooked noodles, seafood mixture, Parmesan cheese and Cheddar cheese in a 9×13×2-inch baking dish. Repeat layer.
5. Bake, on middle oven rack, in a preheated 350°F oven for 45 minutes.

◆ ◆ ◆

Spinach Lasagne

(SERVES 16)

This was Jeff's favourite vegetarian lasagne recipe. It is full of antioxidants from the spinach, tomatoes and mozzarella cheese. A green salad is the perfect accompaniment to this meal.

Leftover lasagne is best kept in a covered container in the refrigerator for 2 to 3 days. It can be reheated in the microwave the next day. This recipe freezes well in freezer containers for up to 3 months.

16 lasagne noodles

boiling water

dash of extra virgin olive oil (antioxidant)

all-purpose cooking spray (or 1 tablespoon olive oil)

2 medium onions, peeled and chopped (antioxidant)

4 × 10 oz/284 mL cans sliced mushrooms, drained well

2 × 15 oz cans all-purpose tomato sauce (antioxidant)

2 × 5½ oz/156 mL cans tomato paste (antioxidant)

1½ teaspoons dried oregano leaves

salt, to taste

⅛ teaspoon dried basil leaves

4 cups/1 kg 2% cottage cheese

2 large eggs, beaten (antioxidant)

2 × 300 g packages frozen chopped spinach, thawed, drained and
squeezed dry (antioxidant)

freshly ground black pepper, to taste

¾ cup Parmesan cheese, grated

340 g package part-skim mozzarella cheese, shredded (antioxidant)

1. Fill a large pot with enough water to cover noodles. Bring water to a boil over high heat.
2. Cook noodles with olive oil, uncovered, about 15 minutes. Drain and set aside.
3. Spray the bottom of a large pot with all-purpose cooking spray.
4. Cook onions over medium heat for 3 to 4 minutes until softened.

5. Stir in mushrooms, tomato sauce, tomato paste, oregano, salt and basil. Cook another 12 to 13 minutes. Set aside.

6. Combine cottage cheese, eggs, spinach and black pepper in a bowl. Set aside.

7. Layer ½ noodles, ½ mushroom sauce, spinach mixture, remaining ½ noodles and mushroom sauce, Parmesan cheese and mozzarella cheese on top in a 12¼×10½×2½-inch baking dish.

8. Spray a sheet of aluminum foil with cooking spray. Cover lasagne with greased foil.

9. Bake, on middle oven rack, in a preheated 350°F oven for 1 hour. Then remove foil and broil in oven for 5 to 6 minutes to brown cheese on top.

◆ ◆ ◆

Vegetarian Pasta Salad

(SERVES 8)

This quick pasta recipe is perfect for the summer months when you do not want to spend much time in a hot kitchen. It is also loaded with antioxidants.

Leftover pasta salad is best kept in a covered container in the refrigerator for up to 3 days.

2¼ cups rotini (corkscrew pasta twists), cooked according to package directions and drained well

2 cups mozzarella cheese, cubed ½-inch (light preferred) (antioxidant)

3½ cups broccoli crowns, cut into bite-size pieces (antioxidant)

1 medium red bell pepper, cut into bite-size chunks (antioxidant)

¼ cup canola oil

¼ cup pure apple cider vinegar

1 tablespoon white granulated sugar

1 teaspoon dried oregano leaves

¾ teaspoon dried basil leaves

freshly ground black pepper, to taste

1. Combine cooked pasta, cheese, broccoli and red pepper in a large salad bowl.
2. Mix together remaining ingredients in a small bowl. Drizzle dressing over salad and toss gently to coat well.
3. Cover and refrigerate at least 2 to 3 hours before serving.

◆ ◆ ◆

Chicken and Shrimp Fried Rice

(MAKES 8 CUPS)

This healthy dish makes a complete meal for all occasions and is loaded with antioxidants. It can be halved, if desired.

Leftovers can be stored in a covered container in the refrigerator for 2 to 3 days. They can be reheated in the microwave. This recipe freezes well in freezer containers for up to 2 months.

2 tablespoons canola oil

1½ lbs skinless and boneless chicken, cubed ¾-inch

½ lb cooked shrimp

1½ teaspoons extra virgin olive oil (antioxidant)

6 large eggs, beaten (antioxidant)

salt, to taste

black pepper, to taste

1 tablespoon extra virgin olive oil, extra (antioxidant)

¾ cup sliced celery (antioxidant)

2 cups sliced mushrooms

4–4½ cups cold cooked rice (antioxidant)

3–4 tablespoons dark soy sauce

2 cups frozen green peas, partially thawed

3 chopped green onions (antioxidant)

¾–1 cup chicken broth

1. Heat canola oil in a large saucepan over medium heat. Cook chicken about 4 minutes until meat is no longer pink inside. Add shrimp and cook another 1½ minutes. Set aside.

2. Heat 1½ teaspoons olive oil, salt and pepper in a skillet over medium heat. Cook eggs, without stirring, for 1½ minutes on each side. Cut into shreds with a sharp knife. Add to chicken and shrimp. Set aside.

3. Heat 1 tablespoon olive oil in a large saucepan. Cook celery and mushrooms over medium heat until tender. Add rice, soy sauce, peas, onions and chicken broth. Stir well.

4. Add chicken and shrimp mixture. Cook and stir for a few minutes until heated.

◆ ◆ ◆

Prawn, Crab and Avocado Sushi

(MAKES 8 LARGE ROLLS)

This Asian recipe is perfect as an appetizer or light meal. This recipe can be halved, if desired. Sushi is best eaten fresh.

6 cups short/medium grain sushi rice, washed, drained and
  let stand 20 minutes

⅔ cup Japanese rice vinegar

2 tablespoons white granulated sugar

1 tablespoon salt

1½ lbs cooked prawns

2 packages imitation crab (or 2 × 4 oz/120 g cans drained crabmeat)

½ long English cucumber, washed and sliced lengthwise

2 medium ripe avocados, cut into 16 wedges (antioxidant)

Wasabi paste (optional)

8 sheets dried nori seaweed

Japanese rice vinegar, extra

1. Combine prepared rice with 6 cups of water in a large saucepan. Cover and bring to a boil over high heat. Then reduce heat to medium-low and simmer 20 to 25 minutes until water is all absorbed. Let stand for 20 minutes. Pour cooked rice into a large bowl.

2. Combine vinegar, sugar and salt in a medium saucepan. Cook over high heat until sugar dissolves. Pour over rice and fold in mixture. Cool rice to room temperature.

3. Place flat, non-textured and shiny side of nori down on bamboo rolling mat. Cover sheet with cooked rice, within 1 inch from edges. Layer prawns, crab, cucumber and then avocado slices on top. Wet end of nori sheet with additional rice vinegar to seal each roll. Cut each roll into 8 slices with a sharp knife dipped in water each time.

◆ ◆ ◆

Rice Casserole

(SERVES 6)

This simple recipe is perfect as a side dish.

Leftover casserole is best stored in a covered container in the refrigerator for 2 to 3 days. It can be reheated in the microwave.

1½ cups long grain rice, rinsed and drained (antioxidant)

1 × 10 oz/284 mL can sliced mushrooms, drained well

2 × 10 oz/284 mL cans beef broth

3 tablespoons margarine

1. Combine all ingredients together in a large casserole dish.
2. Bake, on middle oven rack, in a preheated 350°F oven for 1 hour, stirring halfway through baking time.

◆ ◆ ◆

Spanish Rice

(SERVES 6–8)

This recipe is loaded with antioxidants and perfect as a side dish.

Leftovers can be stored in a covered container in the refrigerator for 2 to 3 days. They can be reheated in the microwave.

all-purpose cooking spray

1 medium green bell pepper, seeded and chopped (antioxidant)

1 small onion, peeled and chopped (antioxidant)

1 cup long grain rice, rinsed and drained (antioxidant)

2 cups canned tomatoes, cut up, with juices (antioxidant)

2 cups water

salt, to taste

black pepper, to taste

1. Spray the bottom of a large saucepan with all-purpose cooking spray.
2. Cook green pepper and onion over medium heat for 2 to 3 minutes.
3. Add rice and cook until golden brown, stirring constantly, for 10 to 13 minutes.
4. Add tomatoes, water, salt and black pepper. Cover. Reduce heat to medium-low and simmer 30 to 35 minutes until water is all absorbed and rice is flaky.

◆ ◆ ◆

VEGETABLES & SAUCE

Vegetables

Sauce

Asparagus Spears with Flax Seed Oil

(SERVES 3–4)

Jeff really enjoyed this healthy and low-fat dish while he was recovering from cancer treatments.

Leftovers can be stored in a covered container in the refrigerator. It is best eaten the next day.

water

½ teaspoon salt

1 lb fresh asparagus spears, bottom trimmed, washed and halved (antioxidant)

1 tablespoon flax seed oil (antioxidant)

1. Fill a large saucepan with enough water to cover asparagus. Add salt. Bring to a boil over medium-high heat.
2. Cook asparagus in boiling salted water for 4 to 5 minutes until cooked but still crisp-tender.
3. Remove from saucepan and transfer to a shallow serving dish.
4. Drizzle with flax seed oil.

◆ ◆ ◆

Curried Potatoes

(SERVES 6)

This vegetarian side dish has the exotic flavour of curry.

This spiced recipe is more suitable for after cancer treatments.

Leftovers can be stored in an airtight container in the refrigerator for 2 to 3 days. They can be reheated in the microwave.

all-purpose cooking spray

6 cups potatoes, peeled, cooked and cut into ¾-inch cubes (antioxidant)

1 small onion, peeled and chopped (antioxidant)

6 tablespoons all-purpose flour

1¼ tablespoons curry powder (antioxidant)

freshly ground black pepper, to taste

2½ tablespoons tomato paste (antioxidant)

2 × 10 oz/284 mL cans chicken broth

1. Spray the bottom of a large saucepan with all-purpose cooking spray.
2. Cook onion over medium heat for 2 to 3 minutes.
3. Stir in remaining ingredients, except potatoes until well mixed. Cook and stir until thickened.
4. Add potatoes and pour mixture into a large casserole dish.
5. Bake, on middle oven rack, in a preheated 375°F oven for about 40 minutes.

◆ ◆ ◆

Deep Fried Zucchini Sticks

(SERVES 6)

These zucchini sticks are crisp on the outside and tender on the inside, but they contain extra calories. They are best eaten while still warm.

This recipe can be halved, if desired.

canola oil

3 medium zucchinis, washed and cut into
  ½-inch thick wedges

⅓ cup skim milk (antioxidant)

½ cup all-purpose flour

½ teaspoon salt

¼ teaspoon black pepper

2 large eggs, beaten (antioxidant)

¾ cup fine bread crumbs

1. Combine flour, salt and pepper in a mixing bowl. Set aside.
2. Dip zucchini wedges in milk, followed by flour mixture, then beaten eggs and bread crumbs.
3. Deep fry in hot 375°F oil 3 to 4 minutes on each side until browned.
4. Transfer to a paper-towel lined baking sheet to drain fat.

◆ ◆ ◆

East Meets West Vegetarian Casserole
(SERVES 6–8)

This is a perfect side dish. The water chestnuts and bean sprouts provide a nice crunch.

Leftover casserole can be stored in a covered container in the refrigerator for 2 days. It can be reheated in the microwave.

> 500 g package frozen cut green beans, partially cooked 5 to 6 minutes and drained well
>
> 1 × 7½ oz/227 mL can sliced water chestnuts, drained well
>
> 1 × 28 oz/796 mL can bean sprouts, drained well (or 1 lb fresh bean sprouts, rinsed and drained)
>
> 1 × 10 oz/284 mL can cream of mushroom soup (light preferred)
>
> 1½–1¾ cups light medium Cheddar cheese, grated

1. Layer beans, water chestnuts, bean sprouts, mushroom soup, and then cheese last in a 2-quart or 8-inch square glass baking dish.
2. Bake, on middle oven rack, in a preheated 350°F oven for 35 to 40 minutes.

◆ ◆ ◆

Glazed Carrots

(SERVES 6)

This is a healthy, yet sweet, side dish.

Leftover carrots can be stored in a covered container in the refrigerator for 2 to 3 days. They can be reheated in the microwave.

> water
>
> dash of salt
>
> 6 medium carrots, halved crosswise and cut into 2 or 3 sticks
>   lengthwise (antioxidant)
>
> 1½ tablespoons margarine
>
> ⅓ cup brown sugar
>
> 1 tablespoon fresh parsley, chopped

1. Fill a large saucepan with enough water to cover carrots. Add salt. Bring to a boil over medium-high heat.
2. Cook carrots over medium heat for 10 minutes until crisp-tender. Drain.
3. Add margarine and sugar. Cook and stir over medium-low heat for 10 minutes until sugar is dissolved.
4. Sprinkle chopped parsley on top.

◆ ◆ ◆

Lemon-Parsley Potatoes

(SERVES 4–6)

This is a nice tart side dish for any meal.

Leftover potatoes can be stored in a covered container in the refrigerator for 2 days. They can be reheated in the microwave.

water

salt, to taste

5 medium potatoes (about 1½ lbs), peeled and quartered (antioxidant)

¼ cup margarine

¼ cup fresh parsley, chopped

1 tablespoon fresh lemon juice (antioxidant)

1. Fill a large saucepan with enough water to cover potatoes. Add salt. Bring to a boil over medium-high heat.

2. Cook potatoes in boiling salted water for 15 to 20 minutes until fork-tender. Drain and transfer to a serving bowl.

3. Melt margarine in saucepan. Stir in parsley and lemon juice. Drizzle over potatoes. Stir lightly to coat well.

◆ ◆ ◆

Mashed Potatoes

(SERVES 6–8)

This is a classic side dish for any meal.

Leftovers can be stored in a covered container in the refrigerator for 2 days. They can be reheated in the microwave.

> water
> 6 medium potatoes (about 2 lbs), peeled and cut into
>   large chunks (antioxidant)
> 2 tablespoons margarine
> salt, to taste
> freshly ground black pepper, to taste
> ¼–⅓ cup skim milk (antioxidant)

1. Fill a large saucepan with enough water to cover potatoes. Bring to a boil over medium-high heat.
2. Cook potatoes in boiling water for 15 to 20 minutes until fork-tender. Drain. Add margarine. Mash with a potato masher.
3. Add salt, black pepper and skim milk. Stir until well mixed, light and fluffy.

◆ ◆ ◆

Mashed Sweet Potato Bake

(SERVES 6–8)

This is the perfect sweet side dish for any meal.

Leftovers can be stored in a covered container in the refrigerator for 2 to 3 days. They can be reheated in the microwave another day.

water

6 medium sweet potatoes (antioxidant)

2 tablespoons freshly squeezed orange juice (antioxidant)

2 tablespoons brown sugar

2 tablespoons margarine

salt, to taste

1 large egg, beaten (antioxidant)

½ cup skim milk (antioxidant)

1. Fill a large saucepan with enough water to cover sweet potatoes. Bring to a boil over medium-high heat.
2. Cook whole sweet potatoes for 15 to 20 minutes until fork-tender. Peel and cut up into large chunks before mashing with a potato masher in a large mixing bowl.
3. Add remaining ingredients and beat with a wooden spoon until light and fluffy.
4. Pour mixture into a one-quart casserole dish. Cover with aluminum foil.
5. Bake, on middle oven rack, in a preheated 350°F oven for 50 minutes.

◆ ◆ ◆

Mixed Vegetables with Cashew Nuts
(SERVES 4–5)

This Asian-inspired vegetarian dish is perfect for meatless dinners.

Leftovers can be stored in a covered container in the refrigerator for up to 3 days. They can be reheated in the microwave.

4¼ cups frozen mixed vegetables, partially thawed

1 cup cut baby corn

1 × 10 oz/284 mL can sliced mushrooms, drained well

2 cups fresh white mushrooms, washed and sliced

4 tablespoons oyster sauce

dash of dry sherry

1¼ tablespoons sesame oil

2 tablespoons cornstarch, mixed with ⅓ cup water

1 teaspoon white granulated sugar

1 teaspoon salt

1½ cups roasted salted cashews

hot boiled/steamed rice (antioxidant)

1. Combine all ingredients, except nuts and rice, in a large saucepan.
2. Cook and stir over medium-high heat for 15 to 17 minutes.
3. Sprinkle cashews on top.
4. Serve with hot cooked rice.

◆ ◆ ◆

Cheese Sauce

(MAKES 1 CUP)

This sauce is perfect over any hot cooked vegetables, especially antioxidant-rich broccoli.

Leftover sauce can be stored in an airtight container in the refrigerator for up to 2 days.

2 tablespoons margarine
2 tablespoons all-purpose flour
salt, to taste
black pepper, to taste
1¼ cups skim milk (antioxidant)
1⅛ cups Cheddar cheese, shredded (light preferred)
hot cooked broccoli or cauliflower (antioxidant)

1. Melt margarine in a large saucepan over medium heat.
2. Stir in flour, salt and pepper.
3. Add milk and stir until thickened and bubbly.
4. Reduce heat to low and stir in cheese until melted.
5. Serve with hot cooked broccoli or cauliflower.

◆　◆　◆

INDEX